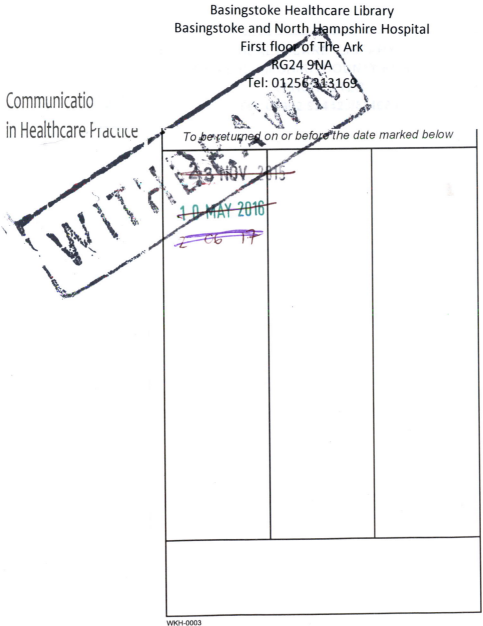
Communicatio
in Healthcare Practice

Communication and Professional Relationships in Healthcare Practice

Sally Candlin and Peter Roger

equinox

Published by Equinox Publishing Ltd.

UK: Unit S3, Kelham House, 3 Lancaster Street, Sheffield, South Yorkshire S3 8AF

USA: ISD, 70 Enterprise Drive, Bristol, CT 06010

www.equinoxpub.com

First published 2013

ISBN   978-1-908049-96-4   (hardback)
            978-1-908049-97-1   (paperback)

British Library Cataloguing-in-Publication Data
A catalogue record for this book is available from the British Library.

Library of Congress Cataloging-in-Publication Data
Candlin, Sally.
  Communication and professional relationships in healthcare practice /
Sally Candlin and Peter Roger.
     pages cm
  Includes bibliographical references and index.
  ISBN 978-1-908049-96-4 (hardback) -- ISBN 978-1-908049-97-1 (pbk.)
 1. Health care teams. 2. Allied health personnel and patient. 3.
Interpersonal communication. 4. Communication in medicine. I. Roger,
Peter, 1964- II. Title.
  R729.5.H4C36 2013
  610.7306'9--dc23
                          2012047616

Typeset by Steve Barganski, Sheffield
Printed and bound in Great Britain by Lightning Source UK Ltd, Milton Keynes,
and Lightning Source Inc., La Vergne, TN

For Chris and Jean
who constantly encouraged us in our work and gave us space
to discuss our ideas and brainstorm in our favourite coffee shop!

Contents

Foreword

The innovative approach taken in this book makes use of adult learning principles to introduce healthcare professionals to theoretical concepts from linguistics and discourse analysis that are pertinent to their professional practice. It sets out to enable the healthcare practitioner and reader to develop the ability to draw upon new understandings about discourse and communication so as to enhance their interactions with both patients and with colleagues in ways that support their clinical and interpersonal goals. The authors consistently encourage the reader to reflect on situations that are familiar from their professional worlds so as to discover for themselves the meaning and relevance of new theoretical concepts. For example, in the early chapters, key concepts such as frame and footing, and key themes such as trust are introduced to the reader by way of selected references and discussion. The value of these concepts for illuminating practice is then illustrated through engaging the reader in the analysis of transcribed authentic and authentic-like professional interactions. As the book unfolds, concepts introduced in early chapters are re-invoked and recycled, and new concepts are introduced so as to enhance understanding of communication and miscommunication in a variety of professional situations. Ultimately, in the final chapter, the reader is encouraged to reflect on their new learning and to consider its relevance to their own day-to-day professional practice.

Refreshingly, the book addresses communication not only in interactions between healthcare professionals and patients, but amongst team members and between healthcare professionals in an array of communicatively challenging real-world contexts. It brings home to the reader the complexity of communication in healthcare, and it offers practitioners many tools for reflecting on their own and others' communicative practices and for enhancing their professional interactions.

Catherine O'Grady

Acknowledgements

This book would not have been written without the help and encouragement of a number of people and we would like to acknowledge and express our gratitude to them for this involvement.

First of all, we thank Janet Joyce and Valerie Hall from Equinox for their patience and understanding during the planning and writing process. Their enthusiasm for this project was unwavering and a source of great encouragement for us. Importantly, they believed, with us, that communication and professional relationships are an integral part of healthcare. But communication in any setting, and particularly in the healthcare setting, does not 'just happen'. It is the result of years of experience and learning, and so we felt encouraged to explore the notion of how healthcare practitioners develop skills in communication so that interactions between patients and professional health carers do not breakdown and healthcare is then maximised. Our own experiences as practitioners and teachers lead us to believe that experiential learning methods, where discourse in the professional environment and clinical setting is the focal point for discovery and learning, enhances the development of such communication skills. Importantly, it results in in-depth learning and encourages the process of self-directed learning.

Thanks are due then to the facilities, colleagues and patients who allowed us to record interactions, all knowing that our aims were to improve communication practice in healthcare settings. We cannot name them for reasons of privacy and to maintain confidentiality, but we thank them anyway and acknowledge our gratitude to them.

We are particularly grateful to the reviewers and to our colleague Dr Louise Collingridge, who, as an audiologist, reviewed the text before submission for publication, and gave many keen insights from the viewpoint of a healthcare professional with an academic background. Thanks are due to Steve Barganski for his input and engagement with the work.

Above all we are indebted to Professor Christopher Candlin who never wavered in his enthusiasm for our work. We benefited from his lifelong passion for applied linguistics and his contribution worldwide to the field over many years, and particularly in the area of health communication. He was generous in his suggestions and in offering constructive criticism of our ideas and our writing. We are immeasurably grateful for his insightful help and encouragement.

Finally, we acknowledge the love and support of our families who have constantly encouraged us and enabled us to see this book through to completion.

About the Authors

Sally Candlin, in her position of Honorary Senior Research Fellow in the Department of Linguistics at Macquarie University, has taught and supervised students in the Masters program in Communication in Professions and Organisations. Her research and writing is within the area of health communication. She has published, nationally and internationally, reports of her research in both nursing and applied linguistic journals. She has been an invited contributor to a number of books, and in 2008 the textbook, of which she was the sole author, *Therapeutic communication: A lifespan approach* was published by Pearson Education (Sydney). She received a BA (Hons) from the University of Lancaster, majoring in linguistics and psychology, and an MSc in Public Health from the University of Hawai'i. For her thesis *Towards excellence in nursing: An analysis of the discourse of nurses and patients*, she was awarded a Doctor of Philosophy from the University of Lancaster. She has taught in undergraduate and postgraduate nursing and health programs at the University of Technology, Sydney, The Hong Kong Polytechnic University and the University of Western Sydney. She is a registered nurse, registered midwife and a health visitor, having practised in the UK before relocating to Australia in 1987.

Peter Roger is a Senior Lecturer in Linguistics at Macquarie University. His teaching spans several Master's degree programs, including Applied Linguistics, Communication in Professions and Organisations, and Speech Pathology. He studied Medicine at the University of Sydney and, after graduating, worked as a medical practitioner for several years before going on to complete a Doctor of Philosophy degree with a thesis entitled *Linguistic diversity and the assessment of aphasia*. For a number of years, he also conducted an annual series of medical English workshops at the University of New South Wales. His research interests include communication in healthcare settings (particularly interpreter-mediated interactions) and the assessment and management of communication disorders in situations of linguistic and cultural diversity. He has published in a variety of journals, including the *Journal of Neurology*, *Brain Injury*, *Aphasiology*, *Neuroradiology*, and the *Asia Pacific Journal of Speech, Language and Hearing*.

Transcription Conventions Followed in this Book

,	comma as distinguished from a hesitation
(.)	second/s of pause as distinguished from a comma as a speech mark
// // // //	overlapping speech
word= =word	where the first person's utterance is immediately followed by the next utterance, i.e. there is no discernible pause between two speakers' turns
wo: :rd	prolonged sound in a word
[*italicised speech*]	explanation/comment
(?)	indecipherable speech
...	portion of speech omitted
<u>word</u>	underlined word/syllable represents emphasised word/syllable

The notation symbols that you will see in the book are adapted from the system proposed by Gail Jefferson and now well established in Conversation Analysis.

Glossary of Terms (as Used in this Book)

coherence
A property of a spoken or written text that refers to whether or not it 'hangs together' on a global level as a meaningful whole. Coherence is created by devices intrinsic to the text itself (see *cohesion*), but also by information and inferences added by the listener or reader.

cohesion
The relationships or links between words, sentences and ideas in a spoken or written text, expressed through various devices that tie these elements together. Cohesion often refers to the links or connections on a local level that assist in achieving *coherence* (see above) on a broader level.

communities of practice (CoP)
'Groups of people who share a concern or a passion for something they do and learn how to do it better as they interact regularly' (Wenger 2006). A CoP consists of people who not only share an interest, but also share a 'practice' (something that they do) and a sense of common goals or purposes. In the domain of healthcare, a CoP may refer to a group of professional practitioners who are bound together by membership of a particular profession or to members of different professions who work as a group or team within a given environment.

contextualisation cues
A term coined by Gumperz (1982) to describe the various surface features of a message through which speakers signal what is 'going on' at a particular moment in an interaction. These cues provide information that allows listeners to interpret the meaning of what is being said by signalling the *frame* (see below) in operation.

conversation analysis (CA)
A method of analysing, in microdetail, elements of talk in a specific interaction without necessarily referring to the history or context of the interaction. CA was developed in the late 1960s and early 1970s by a number of researchers, most notably Harvey Sacks, Gail Jefferson and Emmanuel Schegloff.

critical moments

Significant junctures in an interaction which have the potential to upset the status quo, and as a consequence demand appropriate professional attention to restore the balance, or to capitalise on the moment to steer the interaction in a way that assists in achieving the goals of the encounter.

discourse

Discourse can be defined in several different ways. The simplest definition of the term is any stretch of language longer than one sentence. However, the study of discourse generally goes 'behind' the language (the words and syntax) and includes the influence of the total situation on a given communicative event. In this sense, discourse refers to 'language in use, as a process which is socially situated' (C. Candlin 1997: viii). The term 'discourse' can also be used to refer collectively to a whole body of communication types, events and genres associated with a particular professional or social practice (e.g. medical discourse, legal discourse).

discourse analysis

An umbrella term that encompasses a variety of techniques and approaches for examining samples of language in use, or *discourse* (see above). The approach adopted in a given situation depends upon the aims of the analysis (e.g. power relationships, development of trust) as well as the level(s) of focus (e.g. the interaction, the institution or the broader society) that a particular researcher has.

empathy

The capacity to recognise or grasp the way in which another person feels or experiences a particular situation, and (to a certain degree) to share these feelings (cf. *sympathy*).

expertise

An accumulated body of knowledge and skill in a particular area or field that distinguishes a person (the 'expert') from others who do not possess this level of knowledge and skill in the field.

face

The public self-image that an individual wants to claim for himself or herself, consisting of two related aspects: (a) negative face: the basic claim to territories, personal preserves, rights to non-distraction, i.e. to freedom of action and freedom from imposition; (b) positive face: the positive consistent self-image or 'personality' (crucially including the desire that this self-image be appreciated and approved of) claimed by interactants (Brown and Levinson 1987: 61).

facework

Any communication behaviour that is directed to maintaining (or mitigating a possible threat to) the speaker or hearer's positive or negative face (see *face* above).

frames and framing

A frame (or sometimes 'interactive frame') refers to 'what is going on' at any given moment in an interaction. A shared understanding of the frame in operation at any moment is necessary for participants to be able to interpret the messages (verbal and non-verbal) of the other participants. For instance, the statement 'That's a poor excuse!' from one work colleague to another would be interpreted very differently in a 'joking' frame and an 'arguing' frame.

hedges

Language features that allow us to express ideas in tentative or less-than-certain terms. The use of such features to express various degrees of possibility or probability is called 'hedging'.

impression

The way in which individuals present themselves and their activities to others (Goffman 1959).

impression management

Actions (which are often, but not always, verbal actions) that are directed at controlling the *impression* that one presents to others in the course of interacting with them.

institution

Refers to a bureaucratic organisation (e.g. a hospital), a profession (e.g. institution of medicine or nursing) or a socio-political entity (e.g. a government department or political party).

interdiscursivity

The idea that *discourses* (see above) influence, and are influenced by, other discourses.

metaphor

The understanding of one idea, concept or process in terms of another. For instance, a company's financial position could be described as 'healthy', 'ailing' or 'terminal', which are all terms used to describe human health and illness. Cameron (2010) argues that metaphor can be viewed as having multiple dimensions, including cognitive, linguistic, affective, embodied, socio-cultural and dynamic.

perspective display sequence	A term used by Maynard to refer to 'a strategy for giving an opinion by first soliciting another party's opinion and then producing one's own report in a way that takes the other's into account' (1989: 91).
politeness	Communicative behaviours and choices that are concerned with saving or maintaining the *face* (see above) of the speaker, hearer or a third party. This definition differs from the common everyday meaning of politeness, which refers more generally to notions of socially correct or desirable behaviour.
sympathy	Feelings of compassion for the plight or situation of another person (cf. *empathy*).
total situation focused approach (TSF)	A concept which is described as: 'a situation where the healthcare practitioner (in *this* context – but could be adapted to any social context) not only recognises the person's physical, social, emotional and spiritual needs, but also understands the total situation: the meaning of the situation not only for the individual but also for the society of which the patient is a member. The situation is a state which in turn requires the healthcare practitioner to understand the wider ramifications: the socio-political and economic forces, the community situation and needs, and cultural factors – what might be termed an ecological approach to care or total situation focused healthcare ...' (S. Candlin 1997b: 19 (adapted)).

Introduction to the Book

How this book came about

This book arose from our experiences as healthcare professionals in the respective fields of nursing and medicine, and from an early realisation of the centrality of discourse in our professional practice. This realisation was later re-enforced by our research activities in the area of health communication, and these in turn informed our work with students, a number of whom were healthcare professionals studying in the Master of Communication in Professions and Organization (MACPO) programme in the Department of Linguistics at Macquarie University. We were conscious of the contribution which linguistics and discourse analysis as a field of study could make in raising awareness in students of the complexities of communication, not only between health professionals and patients, but also between healthcare professionals from the different disciplines. This awareness developed into a quest by our students to fill what some perceived to be a gap in their knowledge base which might be met by studies in a field other than their practice specialty. The new knowledge gained we (and they) believed could be applied to their existing knowledge and professional and life experiences to enhance their professional practice.

Acknowledging and applying principles of adult learning

In developing the programme, we were aware that students with considerable life and professional experience had much to contribute to their own and to each others' learning experiences. Adopting adult learning principles, where students are encouraged to be autonomous learners identifying their own learning needs, ensured that the curriculum was practically and motivationally relevant to each individual student. We took an experiential approach to gathering and analysing information where extracts of discourse which related to theoretical concepts were analysed, drawing upon our own and students' practice experiences. This is an approach we have followed in this book.

Developing materials which contributed to learning and would guide research activities

Our research and teaching raised our awareness of a need for a book which could be made available both to those unable to access formal face-to-face study programmes, as well as one which could be useful for those pursuing postgraduate study in distance mode, such as in continuing education programmes. This book is the result and has its genesis in the practice experiences of healthcare professionals.

It consists of twelve chapters with the first three concentrating on theoretical underpinnings of communication, together with an introduction to methods of analysis of interactions. These initial chapters are followed by others which address some of the concepts experienced in everyday situations, such as, for example, demonstrations of empathy and sympathy, issues of face, assertiveness, aggression, conflict, the breaking of bad news and how such situations are, and can be, managed in the discourse of the participants in clinical situations. We examine concepts such as the identification and achievement of professional, social and discoursal goals – how we construct our discourse to achieve these goals, whether we are in a 'one-to-one' situation with a patient or another health professional, or in multidisciplinary team meetings. Each chapter introduces theoretical underpinnings of those discourse situations which are then illustrated by means of extracts of authentic data (gathered mainly from research activities), or simulated situations which have been informed by experience. Further, each chapter affords opportunities for the reader to reflect on their learning. These allow and encourage readers to consider the possible application of learning to professional and life experiences. We believe that this approach can enhance understanding, not only of new learning but, importantly, of professional practice.

How to use this book

This book, as with our teaching, has been written so that independent readers/ learners or those in taught courses will be able to engage in a rich learning environment and draw considerable benefit from the study of concepts which might be novel to them.

As we indicated above, each chapter intersperses theoretical underpinnings with opportunities for you to reflect on authentic and simulated discourse situations. In this way, we hope that you, the reader, will be enabled to appreciate the relevance of theory to practice, one underpinning and informing the other. Each chapter has been written as a discrete unit, but by referring to other chapters which are indicated in the text, and by drawing on the index and the glossary of terms, you can study any chapter in no particular order, constructing your own ways of using the book. So, while each chapter – particularly the first three – emphasises analytical methods, you do not have to read and study them sequentially.

You can use this book as an independent learner if you are unable conveniently to access teachers and other resources. Equally, teachers can use the book to augment their own programmes. Groups of like-minded professionals can use it as a book which will guide your approach to understanding principles of communication. You might then be stimulated to embark on research activities related to professional practice, so that your practice may be enhanced.

The essence of the book is that theoretical principles are set out in each chapter, followed by authentic, or sometimes simulated, extracts of discourse. To help you build up your own bank of resources, some chapters include a section which indicates further useful readings. The final chapter brings together concepts from the book; by constructing your own framework related to your reading, learning and practice, we hope that you can make your knowledge practically and motivationally relevant.

1   A Framework for the Study of
        Interactions in Healthcare Settings

Concepts to be introduced, explored and applied

- What is discourse?
- What is communication? An introduction to explanatory models
- An overview of communication in workplace environments
- Adult learning principles

Objectives of this chapter
After completing the study of this chapter you will be able to:

- identify the differences between discourse and communication;
- analyse models of communication;
- understand the centrality of discourse in professional practices.

1.1   Introductory discussion of key concepts

1.1.1   An approach to learning

The overall aim of this book is to develop your professional communication skills. You may already have considerable understanding of aspects of communication practices – perhaps much of it intuitive. The objectives of this book are to enable you to build upon this knowledge and apply it to professional sites, particularly in healthcare situations.

Taking the adult learning approach central to this book, you are encouraged to become independent learners, where you will engage in a process of discovery, identifying what you already know as well as the areas where you need to develop your knowledge further, and then apply a set of developing skills and strategies in your professional practice. To this end, each chapter will consist of discourse-based interactions set in a healthcare context. The approach we are taking is not 'didactic' but one where you are presented with situations which will lead you into a deeper understanding of discourse and communication skills. As adult learners, you will draw upon life and professional experiences to address situations which may or may not be problematic – for you as a learner or for the healthcare team and the patient – but they will raise interesting challenges. We are not therefore concerned with 'solving' health-related problems, but determining how the study and use of discourse can be focused to help us improve how we work in a range of relevant situations. This means, above all, considering not just the multidisciplinary team, but the patient, family and the wider psychosocial setting: in fact, what we refer to in this book as a *total situation focused* approach to learning (TSF). This is a concept which is described as:

> a situation where the *healthcare practitioner* not only recognises the person's physical, social, emotional and spiritual needs, but also understands the total situation – the meaning of the situation[1] not only for the individual but also for the society of which the patient is a member. The situation is a state which in turn requires the healthcare practitioner to understand the wider ramifications of the situation – the socio-political and economic forces, the community situation and needs, and cultural factors – what might be termed an ecological approach to care or *total situation focused healthcare...* (S. Candlin 1997b: 19 (adapted)).

In this book, therefore, we consider the total situation to include the discrete elements of discourse, how they can be integrated, and how they are applied.

You will be guided in your learning by studying scenarios which ask you to reflect on a given situation represented by the discourse of participants, approaching it by first identifying what you already know and then what you need to know. You are given no information other than a brief introduction to a situation, represented in an extract of discourse taking place in a workplace context. You will need to generate hypotheses about aspects of this situation. For example: how will you find information which will help in your learning and improve your knowledge base so that you understand the situation better? If you

---

[1] The situation includes of necessity the discourse practices of the healthcare practitioners as an integral component of healthcare.

are studying with other colleagues, then discussion of the situation is the first place to start, followed by a library and/or online search for information. Additionally, you will need to consult your facilitator and explore recommended texts for further reading. This will help you reflect on your learning and practice experiences.

To consolidate your learning, there will follow a commentary based on the objectives of the chapter, which will then further guide your learning by presenting you with an opportunity to reflect on your learning in the light of insights gleaned from the commentary. This might, for example, take the form of series of prompts which you may not have already addressed – or even perhaps thought of!

1.2   An approach to understanding the complexity of the communication process

1.2.1   What is discourse?

When we talk or write with another person we engage in discourse, a concept which is much broader and deeper than language. It is more than just speaking or writing a string of words. Discourse, in a sense, goes 'behind' the language (the words and syntax). It considers the impact which the total situation has on what we say, and how we understand and respond to the message that we hear or read. It implies, for example, a consideration of the other person's situation – 'where they're coming from' – and what sort of response you expect and/or want. By way of introduction you might like to consider Figure 1.1 below, which provides a framework for describing and explaining the discourse of professional relationships. We see that central to the discourse of a particular situation is, of course, the professional relationship. Although we are concerned chiefly with healthcare situations and health professionals, the same process applies whatever the professional site, and regardless of the professional participants. These relationships develop and take place in a particular context, at a particular time and place, and involve often very diverse people of different genders and ages, and with their own personalities. They each have come from a specific socio-economic background and have received an education and/or a professional training. They have each developed their own system of values and beliefs. None of these factors can be divorced from the discourse which they produce and in which they engage. It is represented in the following model which you may wish to study.

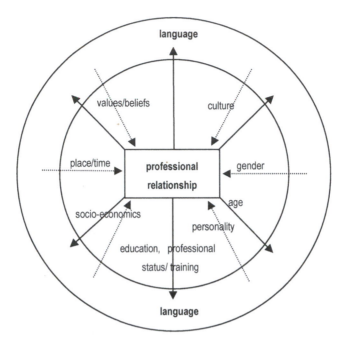

Figure 1.1   The context of professional relationships

Reflective learning 1.1: Professional relationships

Reflect on your professional relationships by critically analysing the model represented in Figure 1.1 and focusing on the prompts below.

- Add any factors to it, or delete what you cannot agree with, and make considered changes both to the factors and their inter-relationships. Try to justify your acceptance or rejection of any aspect, and any other changes that you might wish to make.
- How do you think that each of these factors contributes to your discourse choices, i.e. what you choose to say or write, how you respond, etc.?
- Do people always make the same choices in different situations, for example when speaking or writing to their lovers, parents, children and colleagues? How might the place and nature of the interaction demand different choices?

1.3   The World of Communication model

We will discuss the notion of the discourse process further by analysing another model. Communication is an essential activity upon which all human life depends, and can be represented by the *World of Communication* model below (Figure 1.2). This model demonstrates that communication is not a simple activity as many would believe but is complex in its nature and influenced by many factors. We will analyse this model so that when you consider the interactions which we present in each chapter, you will appreciate in more depth not only how and why people say what they say, but the demands that are made on their discourse, and the effects of the many variables which contribute to individual differences. Underlying these variables are the neuropsychological factors which contribute to the reception and processing of the incoming message, and the psycholinguistic elements which contribute to the production of the response.

1.3.1   Working through the World of Communication model

Beginning at the centre, follow the horizontal line which represents the basic communication process. We find that the message which is received is dependent upon the neurological system, represented in the top half of the inner circle. The message is then processed, and at this point hearers draw upon the way that they perceive the message, but also on their own past life experiences. This all adds up to a particular understanding of the message (Figure 1.3). Therefore, the combined effects of the working neurological system, perception and life experiences allow the hearer to understand the message and can then begin to formulate a response.

Now look at the lower half of the inner circle (Figure 1.4) and you will see that this response may be verbal, non-verbal, visual (e.g. a poster or flyer, an email, a letter) or a combination of these. Clarity is essential if the response message is to be appropriate and effective. When looking at verbal responses, we can examine not only the words (lexis) and grammar (syntax), but also the gap between the 'literal' meaning of the utterance and the speaker's actual meaning (pragmatics). The response may also be partly (or completely) non-verbal, when we make use of non-verbal sounds (e.g. pitch, intonation patterns), or kinesics (body movements), proxemics (use of space) and even exploit the structure of the room. And, if the response (or a component of it) is visual, we need to take account of factors such as typography and design. We need also to consider the hearing ability of the other person, and perhaps think about where the light falls (e.g. on our face and lips), on the way we use our lips and articulate sounds, the way we sit and so forth. The clarity of our response, whether verbal, non-verbal or visual, determines, in part, whether this 'new' message is able to be understood by the interlocutor.

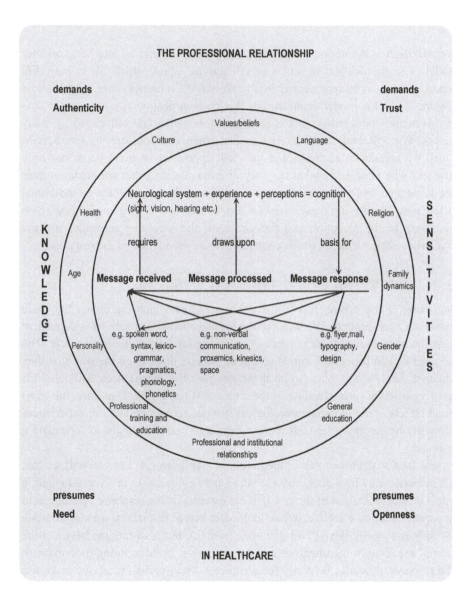

Figure 1.2   The World of Communication (S. Candlin 1992, 2008, extended and adapted)

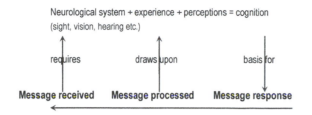

Figure 1.3   The neuropsychological factors underlying the reception
and response of the message

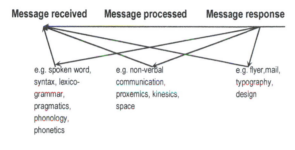

Figure 1.4   The linguistic features of the response

However, participants come to any communicative event with a 'history' which influences both their understanding of a message and the response. These influences we might call *sensitivities*. To what extent are you sensitive to, and aware of the many variables which affect the communication process? Do, for example, age, gender, education, values and/or beliefs affect either the delivery or the reception of the message? These sensitivities are found in the outer circle of Figure 1.2.

Moving now to the space outside of the outer circle, you can see that there are essential elements within a professional relationship in the workplace which must be considered: *trust*, *need*, *openness*, *authenticity*. Of utmost importance is the notion that the interlocutors should be sensitive to the other person and the individual's knowledge base.

Under the umbrella of *healthcare interactions* it is necessary to consider the context or setting, i.e. the type of workplace. For example, is a healthcare setting the patient's home, the recovery room following surgery, the occupational therapy department or some other specialist location? Is the context one of patient education, undergoing a painful procedure, or counselling? Figure 1.4 illustrates the *modalities* which might be used: spoken or written genres, verbal and/or non-verbal communication. Factors such as lexical and syntactic choices, intonation patterns, whether we are dealing with formal letters, reports, publications, flyers and posters (to name a few) all have to be taken into account. These factors and elements are summed up in the **World of Communication** model above and in particular in Figure 1.4 **The linguistic features of the response**.

Reflective learning 1.2: About Figure 1.2

Some texts that address the communication process simply offer a linear model (message received, message processed, message response).

- Critique the the World of Communication model. What can you add to it, for example to the circle of sensitivities? Are there factors which are not accounted for, or are there factors which you think may be unnecessary?
- This is a proposed universal model. Does it apply to healthcare contexts such as your workplace?

1.4   Applying your learning to practice situations

Now we are ready to think about the overall effects which situations and life in general might have on both the client/patient and the professional. The discourse in the scenario presented below (Interaction 1.1) is very complex, but not unusual in the healthcare situation where a number of health professionals are involved in caring for the person.

Reflective learning 1.3: Applying a theoretical model to a practice situation

To ensure that the outcomes of discourse events are successful, speakers and listeners must attend to a number of factors.

Study the transcript of the conversation of the participants in Interaction 1.1 in the light of your reading and what you have learned so far. What specific elements of the World of Communication model, and that of Professional Relationships are illustrated by the way that colleagues communicate in the following interaction?

Interaction 1.1

See Table of transcription symbols (page xiv) to explain transcription symbols used here.

The multidisciplinary team in the Department of Aged Care at St James Hospital is meeting for its weekly case conference. The team consists of the consultant geriatrician (Dr Tony Diaz), registrar (Dr David Bowen), nurse consultant (Jenny Fogerty), physiotherapist (Anne McEnroe), occupational therapist (Jodie Curnow) and speech pathologist (Elisabeth Carter). They are discussing the care of Mr Delaney, who was admitted during the night via the Emergency Department, presenting with a history of headache, slurring of speech and weakness of the left side.

1 Consultant:	We've now come to the new patients. David you were on call last
2	night. Tell us about Mr Delaney.
3 Registrar:	Yes, well Mr Delaney came in early this morning. He's 68, a recently
4	retired financial planner, previously well apart from a history of
5	hypertension. He fell when he got up to go to the bathroom last night
6	and his wife noticed some oddities in his speech. Fortunately she
7	called an ambulance and they brought him straight here. He had a BP
8	reading of 180/90 on arrival, with a left hemiparesis, dysarthria and
9	what looked like an expressive dysphasia as well. The CT in
10	Emergency showed no haemorrhage, so he had intravenous tPA as
11	per the protocol. He's been on anti-hypertensives for a number of
12	years, but by all accounts was otherwise healthy.
13 Consultant:	OK so what investigations have you ordered?
14 Registrar:	Ah.. an MRI, chest x-ray, blood profile an//d//
15 Consultant:	//O//K. Don't suppose
16	anybody else has seen him apart from the nurses. Jenny what can you add?
17 Nurse consultant:	Well he's feeling pretty sick and confused at the moment. He's not
18	eaten much, his swallowing's not good, he's nauseous, incontinent, takes
19	two to lift. His left arm's oedematous and all up he's not a well man.
20 Consultant:	Hmm lot of work ahead here. I'll see him after the conference and then
21	I want to talk with his wife. Anne you'll be doing an assessment today
22	won't you?
23 Physiotherapist:	Yes. I want to see how soon we can check his balance so we can plan
24	his program.
25 Speech pathologist:	Yes and I want to know what his swallowing reflex is like, see if we
26	need nasogastric feeding. I'd like to see Mrs Delaney too, she must be
27	pretty distressed about his speech. See how soon we can get her
28	working with us.
29 Consultant:	Right, who's next Jenny? How's Mrs Smith doing?

1.5   Reflection and problem solving

Before you consider Reflective learning 1.4, ask yourself the following questions:

What do I know? i.e. What are the communication issues that I can identify? (Why do you think is it important that we understand something about the interlocutors (i.e. participants) when considering workplace communication?)

What do I already know: (a) about the work lives of these people, as presented so far, and (b) from my own accumulated life/professional experiences and body of knowledge?

What do I need to know to understand this particular communicative event?

How will I find out? (Colleagues? Tutors? Readings? Other sources?)

How are the communication issues that I have identified relevant to my own workplace?

Reflective learning 1.4: About Interaction 1.1

What considerations must participants make in terms of each of their colleagues, for example in terms of their unique body of professional knowledge and their understanding of the unique body of professional knowledge of their interlocutor?

- Do participants appear to demonstrate awareness of each other's professional boundaries in their plans for care of the patient?
- Discuss the contributions and responses of each of the team members. Would you as a health professional respond differently? For example, would you add more information, be more/less explicit, use different words or sentence structures?
- How might the discourse style change when healthcare professionals talk with patients, rather than with professional colleagues? Interaction 1.2 below is an example of a nurse-patient encounter. If you compare Interactions 1.1 and 1.2 in terms of the words used (i.e. lexical choices), what differences do you notice? What other aspects of discourse style also change?

Interaction 1.2

The following extract of discourse is taken from the conversation between a community nurse visiting a patient in her home.

1 Jane:	Thank you for taking part in this research today. We're just going to be
2	talking about you (...) and how you are, how you manage at home that
3	sort of thing. We've been coming to you for some months now haven't we?
4 Mrs C:	Yes
5 Jane:	Helping you with your showering. You're starting to feel better
6	about that now aren't you?
7 Mrs C:	Oh yes feeling more confident too.
8 Jane:	Mm that's good
9 Mrs C:	But as I say you now if I didn't feel well I wouldn't //have
10 Jane:	//that's right, you're
11	better off not to on those odd days and you're sure there's a nice support in
12	the shower with the rail and all that in it
13 Mrs C:	Yes
14 Jane:	And the rubber mat now that you've//got//
15 Mrs C:	//my//stick has been in the kitchen for
16	two days not used=
17 Jane:	=right so you're becoming stronger//that's// good isn't it
18 Mrs C:	//yes//

1.6   Commentary

From this conversation between a nurse and a patient it appears that they know each other. The nurse is aware of the patient's health history, referring to the patient's general health, her mobility and consequent daily living needs (lines 2, 3, 5, 6). The patient acknowledges the nurse as a professional and discloses information that is pertinent to the nurse's assessment of her health (lines 7, 9, 15, 16). There is no evidence that either the patient or the nurse has any deficits of their neurological systems (see the upper semicircle of the World of Communication model, Figure 1.2). They both draw upon their perception and understanding of the situation – Mrs C's health history and needs, and Jane's provision of professional care, resulting in both of them understanding the other's contribution to the conversation, for example Jane's health-related questions, statements and acknowledgements of Mrs C's responses (see the central line showing the processing of the message). On this understanding, they make their verbal responses (in this extract there is no indication of their non-verbal behaviours) each of which is heard by the other, then processed and a further response made.

However, the responses demonstrate a sensitivity to a number of features, not least of which are Mrs C's health and Jane's education and training.

Reflective learning 1.5: Applying a theoretical model to an interaction

Reflect on the above explanation of Interaction 1.2.

- Are there any other identifiable factors which you can add to this, e.g. features to which either participant is sensitive?
- The above extract of discourse (Interaction 1.2) is of course different in many aspects from the first extract (Interaction 1.1). This is a conversation between just two people, and only one is a health professional, while the first extract is discourse produced by a number of professional people. Can you identify any other differences? Can you suggest how these differences might affect the discourse?
- If the situation was one which did not involve healthcare, i.e. the participants were two acquaintances, how might the conversation have differed? Give some reasons for this. Can the circle of sensitivities explain any differences in the discourse?

From insights gathered as a result of your reading and discussion, consider again Interaction 1.1 between the members of the healthcare team in the Department of Geriatric Medicine.

- What does the discourse tell us about their working and professional relationships (who, for example, appears to lead the team)?
- How does the discourse reflect their concerns about the current situation?
- As a result of the commentary offered on the extract of discourse between Jane and Mrs C would you make changes to your discussion in Reflective learning 1.4?

1.7   Discussion: issues to consider in the application of discourse concepts

As we have presented concepts which are possibly new to you, you have been encouraged to reflect on the discourse of conversations (or interactions) in a different light. You may or may not have previously given much consideration to the complexities of our interactions, or the impact of factors such as age, gender, education, sociocutural aspects have on the way we talk to and understand each other – our interlocutors. In your reflections, have you, for example, considered the following issues:

- How does each participant *enter* the conversation in these interactions?
- What are some of the ways in which people typically 'open' or enter conversations in your own workplace?
- What are some of the factors that might influence how this is done? How does this differ from the home/ social situation?
- Can you make any comments about how people *change topics*? For example, in this extract of data between nurse and patient does one participant change the topic more often than the other? Does the discourse behaviour differ from that of the discourse behaviours in the group of professionals?
- In a different setting, how do you suggest that these scenarios might be played out? Can you identify, from your own experiences, differences between professional and social situations, e.g. between a work situation and a family group or a group of friends?
- Identify the different agendas of the participants in both extracts of data. How are they being enacted, i.e. what communication strategies do participants use to achieve their goals?
- Can you apply any of the concepts you considered in relation to the World of Communication model? Are there aspects of the model which do or do not explain the discourse behaviours of the family members?

These are issues which you may not have considered but will surface as you work through later chapters

1.8   Summary

In this chapter we have considered some theoretical models of communication and considered the complexities of the communication process, reflecting on the application of these models to professional practices. You have briefly analysed extracts of discourse taking a TSF approach, and have also discussed the role of independent learning and exploration as a means of enhancing our learning. In the next chapter, we will examine some specific features of discourse which will help you understand specific discourse behaviours, for example how participants take turns at talking. In Chapter 2, then, we introduce you to conversation analysis, a method of analysing conversations which is concerned with the local situation, i.e. the management of the discourse, rather than the wider situation and the impact of sociocultural and relational aspects. The analysis considers how conversations are managed: who 'holds the floor' and how participants 'enter' the conversation and take turns to speak, how sequences of turns are structured, and how topics of conversation are managed. We will then consider further issues which add to the complexities of the communication process when you reflect on the way you talk with others.

Further reading

Boud, D. and Felletti, G. (eds.) (1997). *The challenge of problem-based learning*, 2nd edn. London: Kogan Page.

Schön, D. (1987). Changing patterns in inquiry in work and living. *Journal of the Royal Society of Arts Proceedings* 135: 225-31.

2   Managing the Interaction

Concepts to be introduced, explored and applied
Conversation analysis in the management of interactions:

- Opening and closing conversations
- Sequences of interactions
- Topic control
- Turn-taking
- Repairs and clarification

Objectives of this chapter
After completing the study of the issues addressed in this chapter
you will be able to:

- identify and understand theoretical issues through the analysis
  of data from sites of engagement;[1]
- apply theoretical insights to professional practice situations;
- identify strategies used for the successful management of interactions;
- understand some of the reasons why conversations break down and
  how such breakdowns can be repaired.

2.1   Introduction

This chapter introduces, explores and applies concepts related to the management
of interactions in the healthcare workplace, and how these interactions differ
from those in other social settings. Interactions in particular environments, such

---

[1] Sites of engagement refer to specific sites where activities and discourses related to that site
occur.

as institutional settings or ordinary everyday conversation can be thought of as different *speech exchange systems*, a concept of which you should be aware since these differing systems affect, for instance, how turns in the interaction are allocated to different speakers. For example, in an interview situation, the topics of conversation and the speaking turns of participants are under the control of the interviewer(s), the interviewee having very little legitimate/licit control of the interaction. Similarly, in a court of law there are set procedures for who is allowed to speak. You might consider how these and other institutional settings (e.g. news conferences, debates, doctor–patient interactions, traditional church services) differ from ordinary day-to-day conversations. Sacks, Schegloff and Jefferson make the point that:

> [t]he linear array is one in which one polar type (exemplified by conversation) involves 'one turn at a time' allocation, i.e. the use of local allocational means; the other pole (exemplified by debate [or ceremony] involves pre-allocation of all turns; and medial types (exemplified by meetings [or classrooms]) involve various mixes of pre-allocational means (Sacks, Schegloff and Jefferson 1974: 729).

Markee (2000) makes the point that where a speech exchange system is more locally managed, there is the potential for many speakers to be treated as 'legitimate' speakers. In such a context this might present a challenge for interlocutors to produce a coherent and co-operative conversation. He also states that such a system is not designed to ensure an equal distribution of turns (p. 87). Where the speech system allows for pre-allocated turns, Sacks et al. conclude that:

> it appears that conversation should be considered the basic form of speech exchange system with other systems on the array representing a variety of transformations of conversation's turn-taking systems to achieve other types of turn-taking systems (Sacks et al. 1974: 730).

You might reflect on, and compare some interactions between friends in a social gathering, and that of a doctor and patient in an out-patient clinic. Can you, for example, identify who holds the power in any of these settings, and how do you think this might be realised in the discourse? (Power is a concept which will be addressed further in Chapter 11). A good way in would be to observe who appears to initiate turns in the conversation and who takes the longer turns. One reason for this focus is that we are particularly interested in the discourse of participants in healthcare – both patients and healthcare practitioners, in the community or hospital[2] – because we believe that the relationships formed and developed through such interactions determine in no small measure both the quality and outcomes of care. Exploring the dynamics and complexities of the discourses of interlocutors, be they doctors and patients, nurses and patients, physiotherapists and patients or between professionals (either inter- or intra-professionally) is one key means by which we can determine the quality of developing relationships.

We are interested in the way that interlocutors *identify goals*, not only *social goals* and the *goals of the activity* in which they are engaged, but also the *discoursal goals* which will facilitate the achievement of both the activity goals and, importantly, the *interactional goals*. Not only can these discoursal and acti-vity goals of healthcare be mutually identified and aligned with by interlocutors (S. Candlin 1997a), but interlocutors also mutually design and structure their talk, that is they *co-construct* their discourse in a spirit of cooperation to identify and achieve those goals. You will be able in this chapter to explore how this cooperation is reflected in the *management of their interactions*, for example: the *control of topics, turn-taking, sequences of turns*, and how *repairs in the discourse* are made and *issues clarified*. The degree of formality in the discourse is also of interest; are some interactions more formal than others, and how does the level of formality in which we choose to express what we want to say affect the relationship? As a way of exploring these and other questions you will consider the interactions of two nurse–patient dyads in health-assessment situations, one taking place in the patient's home and the other in a geriatric rehabilitation unit (Interactions 2.1 and 2.2).

2.2   Application of theory to professional discourse practice

2.2.1   Discourse as a focus for discussion

For learning to be meaningful and useful it needs to be related to reality, in this instance to professional practice within a healthcare setting. Accordingly, this chapter, and the ones that follow, focus on examining authentic or simulated extracts of interactions in healthcare situations. Your task will be to engage in a guided reflection of the texts (see Interactions 2.1 and 2.2) as they relate to key theoretical issues of communication which will in turn help inform your analysis of the discourse.

---

[2] This is not to say that these are the *only* situations where healthcare is delivered.

Interaction 2.1

Nancie, registered nurse, assessing Mrs G's health status in a rehabilitation unit. This is their first meeting.

1 Nancie:	...and when were you born Mrs G
2 Mrs G:	4th of November 1918
3 Nancie::	so your age at the moment is =
4 Mrs G:	=seventy five
	...
46 Nancie:	good now have you had any serious illnesses or
47	disabilities over the last say 20 years
48 Mrs G:	I've had falls and injured myself
49 Nancie:	so you've had a fall //here//
50 Mrs G:	//I had// polio as a child or infantile
51	paralysis it was called
52 Nancie:	right and you were admitted to hospital for that
53 Mrs G:	(?)
54 Nancie:	and you had fractures of your leg
55 Mrs G:	yes unfortunately I have
56 Nancie:	how many have you //had//
57 Mrs G:	//I've// also had muscle injuries that have been
58	attended to by Dr B but he was unable to help me very much but
59	my left leg is still paralysed. I can't (?)
	...

The assessment continues with Mrs G's turns becoming more extended.

341 Nancie:	You've enjoyed your time in Australia at The Beaches? *(an apartment block)*
342 Mrs G:	Yes very much. Sometimes I wish I'd never left U *(her home country)*
343	and people say why don't you go home but then I feel if I go
344	back now after 20 years I wouldn't find the same friends that I had
345	then I only have the one brother and basically I think I'm better off
346	here I think. I have one very good friend here (?) a very
347	kind friend who rings me as I say that's how he found that I'd
348	fallen because we have an arrangement whereby I ring him every
349	morning at eight o'clock and he rings me every night between nine
350	and ten. And I had been lying on the floor since seven thirty and he
351	rang at ten o'clock getting no reply he had the key to my unit and
352	came up to see what was wrong and he ...

Interaction 2.2

Cheryth, a registered nurse assessing health needs of Mrs S following an accident in the garden. This is their first meeting and takes place in the home of Mrs S.

144 Cheryth:	right no other problems no diabetes or heart problems
145	(.) or (.)?=
146 Mrs S:	= I don't know about that. I get breathless at times
147 Cheryth:	right and you've had some high blood pressure
148 Mrs S:	I've got a fair amount of trauma at the moment
149 Cheryth:	What with your blood pressure?
150 Mrs S:	Oh no within the family
151 Cheryth:	Which isn't helping
152 Mrs S:	No
153 Cheryth:	Right so how often would you see your doctor normally to have
154	your blood pressure checked?
155 Mrs S:	Oh I seem to have shot in there on a fairly regular basis for one
156	thing or another. I get these things (?) but I think I've had a lot of
157	depression so I suppose regularly once a month I don't know
158 Cheryth:	But roughly check it about once a month.
159 Mrs S:	Oh easily.
160 Cheryth:	Right and you said you get breathless sometimes.
161 Mrs S:	Yes all of a sudden I'd be talking normally to someone and then I
162	can't get my breath I seem to run out of unless I talk too much
163 Cheryth:	Has the doc have you mentioned to your doctor the breathlessness?
164 Mrs S:	No
165 Cheryth:	And that doesn't isn't a problem in your day to day activities with
166	your housework and things like that?
167 Mrs S:	Oh I don't like playing with the vacuum cleaner. That makes me tired.
168 Cheryth:	Right makes you tired.
169 Mrs S:	Makes me a little breathless yes.
170 Cheryth:	Oh but do you normally do that do you normally do the housework?

Reflective learning 2.1: About Interactions 2.1 and 2.2

Consider how the discourses of the interlocutors in Interactions 2.1 and 2.2 focus on the formality/informality of the individual participants, for example.

- Do the interactions suggest that the discourse in one is more formal than the other? What features in the extracted discourse samples can you identify in support of your response?

2.3   Conversation analysis: a theory to give explanatory value to the organisation of discourse

One important source of information and help in understanding the complexities of interactions and how conversational and social goals may be successfully achieved is the key work of Sacks, Schegloff and Jefferson (1974) in their analysis of conversations, and in the subsequent development of conversation analysis (CA) as an explanatory theory and methodology. CA is an appropriate methodology to draw on since its focus is on the 'here and now' of an interaction, and on the *micro organisation of talk* as it takes place in the interaction. As a consequence, CA is essentially data driven, and analysis of the transcripts of this data[3] can help us determine how talk is co-constructed between the interlocutors.

In this chapter you will explore how the interactions are structured and managed, how topics are controlled in the seeking and giving of information, how turns are taken, and how utterances are repaired as interlocutors seek and offer clarification of their own and their interlocutor's utterances. You might consider too how participants align what they are saying with prior utterances, how they respond to invitations to speak, accepting or declining (usually unspoken) invitations, how they appraise each others turns and how they contribute to the 'deeply ordered, structurally organised social practice' (Hutchby 2007).

In sum we can say that CA is particularly relevant for the examination of health-related discourse since it aims to

> reveal how the technical aspects of speech exchange represent structured, social organised resources by which *participants perform* and *co-ordinate activities through talk-in-interaction* (Hutchby 2007: 20, emphasis added).

CA involves a careful and detailed analysis of the minutiae of talk to show how such talk is mutually designed and structured – it displays an *interaction order*. It is essential therefore that, like Sacks et al., you keep close to the text you are examining and not be sidetracked by the more macro issues of the social and institutional structures – important though they are. (However, as health professionals you will, no doubt, want to be seeing how the text reflects issues of health concern to participants.) Antaki (2011) defines CA as the study of how social action is brought about through the close organisation of talk. The social action you are concerned with is the achievement of healthcare goals, which we have implied is in part best achieved in *cooperative talk* where, together, the interlocutors move the interaction along and contribute to the achievement of

---

[3] Note that the data are the actual conversation and not the transcript of them.

each others' goals – both discoursal and social. The task, then, is to examine professional discourse as something which is mutually constructed and essentially interactive.[4]

In adding to our understanding of CA, Hutchby and Wooffitt state that the aim of CA

> is to reveal the tacit, organized reasoning procedures which inform the production of naturally occurring talk. The way in which utterances are designed is informed by organizational procedures, methods and resources which are tied to the contexts in which they are produced, and which are available to participants by virtue of their membership in a natural language community (Hutchby and Wooffitt 1998: 1).

In their work, then, we find further support for our assertion that CA has utility for our study of interactions in healthcare.

2.3.1   Managing interactions

Some would argue intuitively that conversations are chaotic and 'messy'. Interlocutors *interrupt* each other, and *talk simultaneously*, flouting the belief that there is an implicit rule that:

> only one person speaks at a given moment. Speakers can be distracted by interruptions, they make *false starts* and correct themselves, and each other, giving or asking for clarification i.e. they *repair* conversational errors. However, conversational analysts believe that successful ordinary conversation is not a trivial, random, unorganised phenomenon but a deeply ordered, structurally organised social practice (Hutchby 2007: 20).

Reflective learning 2.2: Messy or rule-governed?

Reflect further on the discourses of the interlocutors in Interactions 2.1 and 2.2 and the discussion presented above.

- From your reading, what instances in the interactions might persuade you that either discourse is 'messy'? What features would you point to which support your view?

(cont.)

---

[4] For further insights into the conduct of interactions you might wish to see the later work of Hutchby (2007), Schegloff (cf. 2007), Drew and Heritage (1992) – particularly in relation to healthcare, and more recently, by such social scientists as Antaki (2011) and Kitzinger (2011).

Reflective learning 2.2 (cont.)

- In contrast, what evidence can you find to support conversation analysts' assertion that discourse is not messy but 'ordered and rule governed'?

These reflections lead us to think further about the management of interactions. The following discussion seeks to develop our understanding of the importance of successful management of conversations.

Firstly, when we enter into a conversation it is often the start or continuation of a relationship, and as such we have certain goals depending upon the situation. For example, we might ask what are our social and discoursal goals when we engage in different everyday activities, such as shopping, planning a social engagement, seeking an appointment with a lawyer etc.? And importantly, for our discussion, we need to determine our social and discoursal goals when we engage in professional practice – be it, for example, in clinical situations, management settings, research or teaching activities. To achieve both social (professional) goals (e.g. the *administering* of medication) and discourse goals (*explaining* the reason for the activity, e.g. the giving of medication, which may involve *giving information*, e.g. about the effects and side effects; *evaluating*, *understanding*) we need to be aware of conduct appropriate to the interaction and to make ongoing judgements related to the discourse as the activity progresses. We size up not only the situation, but also each other, attending not just to what is being said, but to what is *not* being said, and to *non-verbal behaviours*: gaze, facial expression, tone of voice, physical stance etc., how each other acts in relation to interruptions by other people or events, and to the proxemics of the situation and our use of space. Based on these observations, interlocutors make *inferences* about the situation and each other. One of the overriding goals is to judge how engaged the person is with both the event and the interlocutor: the *impressions* we are making on each other (see Chapter 6), how much each person knows about the situation and the people involved, and the trustworthiness and competence of the other person (see Chapter 7). When we study extracts of conversations, we might observe not only how turns are taken, but how participants *orient to the identity* of the other and therefore to the person's needs as well as to the underlying organisation of the activity.

Secondly, we need to be aware of the management of interactions, since if we are unaware of the minutiae of conversations in others then it is difficult to be conscious of our own discourse behaviours and to monitor our discourse strategies to ensure we are achieving goals. We are therefore not looking at discourse in isolation, but considering how the discourse and the situation is impacted by the activity as well as by any extraneous factors – such as the conversations of others in the vicinity. We need also to consider the impact of the discourse on the activity itself. There is then a *symbiotic relationship* between our discourse, the local situation, the wider environment and how each impacts on the other(s): our social relationships, societal institutions and our continuing discourse. To successfully manage interactions, we engage in a 'subset' of discourse behaviours, which include *openings*, *closings* and the overall organisation of the interaction, in particular, the *sequencing of turns* (Sacks et al. 1974).

2.3.2   Openings and closings of conversations

Conversation analysis has described a number of principles which interlocutors orient to in their interactions. Schegloff and Sacks (1973) propose that there are usually clear openings and closings as well as regularities in the intervening conversation. For example, typically a (goal-oriented) telephone conversation begins with a *summons* (bell ringing) followed by a *response* (identification of the speaker and maybe a personal greeting). Then there are formulae for the introduction of the topic and announcement of intent. Within the conversation we might suggest, for instance, a structure similar to the following:

- *Announcements of intent* (e.g. 'Jane I'd like to hear your views on …')
- *Pre-sequences* which prepare the ground for subsequent 'moves' (e.g. a pre-request such as: 'Are you by any chance going to the supermarket?')
- *A pre-announcement* (e.g. 'You'll never guess what happened to Simon.')
- *A pre-closing* (such as 'So to sum up …')
- *Formulations of gist* (e.g. 'So I suppose what's happening here is …')
- *Formulations of upshot* (e.g. 'I'm only telling you this to prepare you for …')

Reflective learning 2.3: Discourse behaviours

> Think of a recent conversation with a patient. Reflect on the structure which utilised any of the above discourse behaviours.
>
> - What was/were your intention/purpose(s)?
> - Why did you select these discourse behaviours in relation to your purpose(s)/intent?
> - What effect/s did your selection have on the interaction? What differences, if any, would you make to how you structure a conversation with a colleague or friend? What factors (e.g. your purpose(s), intent, the situation, etc.) might have an effect on your discourse?

2.3.3   Topic management

In most interactions the conversation does not begin and end with one topic. We digress, we shift from one topic to another, producing a stream of utterances which can result in an animated conversation. In a short space of time we might ask questions, give information, ask for clarification, expand on the original topic, which can lead into another topic, which might throw light on one's views and who we align with. The complexity can be overwhelming. But even in this area there are boundaries. Many of these are determined by our culture, not simply as it relates to ethnicity, but in relation, for example, to the culture of the institution in which the interaction is taking place – of which we may be a member (as a professional carer) or not (as a patient/relative) (see Chapter 1). Relevant questions to think about are:

- Who is allowed to initiate a topic?
- Are there some topics which are permissible depending, for example, on your, or your interlocutor's, sex, age, professional position or social standing?
- How does the choice of topics relate to your goals? And importantly,
- How do we change topics? And in the change,
- How do we ensure that the change, and therefore the interaction, is smooth?

Some changes take place as a result of or making use of what CA refers to as *upshots and formulations*. These are utterances which indicate a need to comment on a previous utterance, sometimes heralded by a discourse marker such as 'so'. Its utility is, for example,

- to confirm/seek confirmation,
- to summarise, or
- to topicalise it; e.g. in Interaction 2.1 Mrs G takes the opportunity to topicalise Nancie's remark about 'enjoying your time in Australia' (line 341) and shifts from emotions about Australia to emotions about her previous home, maintaining the focus on her 'feelings', and thus maintaining the *coherence* (see Chapter 9) of the interaction.

341 Nancie:	You've enjoyed your time in Australia at The Beaches?
342 Mrs G:	Yes very much. Sometimes I wish I'd never left U
343	and people say why don't you go home but then I feel if I go
344	back now after 20 years ...

A speaker may claim the right to formulate or reformulate an utterance, e.g. Cheryth (Interaction 2.2) exercises her power as the healthcare professional to shift the propositional content of line 163, 'breathlessness', to focus on activities of daily living (lines 165–166).

163 Cheryth:	Has the doc have you mentioned to your doctor the breathlessness?	
164 Mrs S:	No	
165 Cheryth:	And that doesn't isn't a problem in your day to day activities with	
166	your housework and things like that?	

Reflective learning 2.4: Topic control

Reflecting on the discussion so far relating to topic control.

- What are some of the topics which, as a health professional, you are privileged to address, but would be inappropriate for a patient to initiate?
- Which of these topics (if any) can you identify in the discourse in Interactions 2.1 and 2.2?

Reflecting on the discussion in this chapter and Chapter 1,

- What might be some of the reasons for the choice of topics? For example, how do they relate to the goals of the interlocutors?
- How might the topics differ in different situations (e.g. if the patient was a child, or the nurse or the patient were of a different gender?)
- How do the interlocutors manage to change topics? That is, what discourse strategies can you identify that speakers use to change the topic? What effect does this have on the listener - and indeed on the course of the interaction?

When one considers the means by which interlocutors shift from one topic to another, a question arises about how topics are selected and who selects them.

- How might speakers indicate that there is to be a change in the topic selection, and how does this contribute to the achievement of conversational and social goals?
- How can the shift be effected seamlessly?

(cont.)

Reflective learning 2.4 (cont.)

Topics in the conversation are selected and controlled: maintained, changed and returned to.

- What topics of conversation can you identify in Interactions 2.1 and 2.2?
- Who appears to determine the topic choice, i.e. the point in the interaction where the topic shifts to another one?

2.3.4   Sequential turns

Following our discussion of how content in interactions is topically organised, we need now to consider how the conversation is structured. As an introduction to the subject of turn-taking in general, we return to our discussion of cooperative conversations, asking whether one particular type of initiating utterance determines the type of the next utterance. Schegloff and Sacks (1973) talk about *adjacency pairs*, i.e. paired utterances where a greeting is followed by another greeting: an offer requires an acceptance, a question requires an answer. The following extracts illustrate such paired utterances.

Illustration 2.1

| 1 Speaker 1 (Nancie): | and when were you born Mrs G? | (Q 1) |
| 2 Speaker 2 (Mrs G): | 4th of November 1918 | (A 1) |

(Question [Q] followed by Answer [A])

Illustration 2.2

| 1 Speaker 1 (Nancie): | You've enjoyed your time in Australia at The Beaches? | (O 1) |
| 2 Speaker 2 (Mrs G): | Yes very much. Sometimes I wish I'd never left U | (A 1, E 1) |

(Offer [O] of a turn followed by Acceptance [A] and, in this case, an extension [E] with the added information 'Sometimes I wish I'd never left U …'

Illustration 2.3

| 1 Speaker 1 (Jo): | How are you? | (Q 1) |
| 2 Speaker 2 (Harry): | Good, and yourself? | (A 1, Q 2) |

(A question/answer sequence - where the response to Q1 is in the form of an answer A1 immediately followed by question Q2, 'and yourself?'

Illustration 2.4

A:	May I have a bottle of wine?	(Q 1)
B:	Are you eighteen?	(Q 2)
A:	No	(A 2)
B:	No	(A 1)

(Levinson 1983: 304)

(Here we can see that there is a second adjacency pair embedded within the first one)

An answer might of course require another response (a comment or a further question as in Illustration 2.3).

In Illustration 2.5 (taken from Interaction 2.2), we can identify another type of sequence where Mrs S is led to a further response resulting not in an adjacency pair, but what we might consider to be a three-part sequence; for example:

Illustration 2.5

148 Mrs S:	I've got a fair amount of trauma at the moment
	(Offer – of information)
149 Cheryth:	What with your blood pressure?
	(Question)
150 Mrs S:	Oh no within the family
	(Answer)

Before reading further, study carefully Interaction 2.2.

- What information does Cheryth need to elicit and clarify?
- Might there be two locations for the second part of an adjacency pair? If so, can you give an example from within the interaction and determine its location in the text?
- From your clinical experiences, identify some examples of adjacency pairs.
- How do they conform (or not) to the order set out by Schegloff and Sacks?

Having thought about the sequence of turns (lines 148–59 taken from Interaction 2.2) we will examine the following four turns in the same interaction (lines 151–55) to clarify our earlier thoughts in Reflective learning 2.2.

Illustration 2.5 (extended)

148 Mrs S:	I've got a fair amount of trauma at the moment
	(Offer – of information)
149 Cheryth:	What with your blood pressure?

	(Question)
150 Mrs S:	Oh no within the family
	(Answer)
151 Cheryth:	Which isn't helping
	(unstated Question)
152 Mrs S:	No
	(Answer)
153 Cheryth:	Right so how often would you see your doctor
154	normally to have your blood pressure checked
	(Complex question)
155 Mrs S:	Oh I seem to have shot in there on a fairly regular basis ...
	(Answer)

Cheryth (in line 151) seems to make a cursory acknowledgment of Mrs S's 'trauma' (referred to in line 148), maintaining a seemingly preferred emphasis on the patient's blood pressure. It is not for another 20 exchanges that the topic of trauma is raised again (referred to as 'a big problem') when Mrs S clarifies the disconnect between 'trauma' (line 148) and 'blood pressure' (line 149).

197 Mrs S:	... and the middle daughter has a big
198	problem at the moment so ...

We can infer that 'the middle daughter' (line 197) relates to 'the family' in line 150.

Reflective learning 2.5: Messiness revisited

After studying the annotation of the extract from Interaction 2.2 above, reflect again on your thoughts in relation to Reflective learning 2.2 and the 'messiness' of interactions.

- Are there perhaps two responses to the issue raised in the reflection related to the messiness or the rule-governed nature of conversations?
- What in fact is going on this interaction? Is there more than one understanding of the topic - and whose interpretation is prioritised? Whose voice then is dominant?

Schegloff and Sacks (1973), when talking about adjacency pairs, say that such pairs are sequences of two utterances that are

1. adjacent,
2. produced by different speakers,
3. ordered as a first part and a second part,
4. typed, so that a particular first requires a particular second, e.g. an offer requires acceptance or rejection.

In Illustration 2.5, we might argue that Mrs S continues in lines 197–98 the response given in line 150 taking the opportunity to add explanation which then affords continuation of talk about her 'trauma'. This would be in line with further discussion by Schegloff and Sacks stating that there are instances when the second part of a pair can indeed come later in the discourse.

Reflective learning 2.6: More on adjacency pairs

Reflecting on conversations you have had with either a colleague or a patient, consider the following:

- How does the concept of adjacency pairs help you understand the organisation of that conversation? Is the notion of adjacency pairs borne out in the conversation?
- What further adjacency pairs can you identify in Interactions 2.1 and 2.2? How are they typed (for example, as offers and acceptances or as questions and answers etc.)? How did interlocutors respond to questions and offers to speak and what were the offers?

2.3.5   Turn-taking

Keeping in mind our main point that participants are essentially cooperative in their discourse and indeed work to co-construct it, we need to look for further evidence. We return to our discussion of topic management and reflect upon the means by which *topics of conversation are selected and controlled*, and how speakers often appear to shift seamlessly from one topic to another. Questions that arise are: who controls the topic choices and the topic exchange, and what discourse strategies are used to effect successful topic control? Addressing these questions will involve examining the *turn-taking* mechanisms within the discourse: when is a turn taken in relation to the previous speaker's turn: who holds the floor and how long is the turn? What are the cues given and understood so that the next speaker's turn is taken appropriately, i.e. without interruption or 'over-talking' the current speaker?

Reflective learning 2.7: Turn-taking

Focus on how turns are managed in Interactions 2.1 and 2.2, i.e. how is a turn passed to the other person? For example, what are the indicators that a turn is finished and then 'offered' to the other person?

- Are there overlaps in the conversation with one person 'over-talking' the other? How are they managed? (For example, does one participant 'give way' to another? How does this affect the interaction?)
- How are the topics changed, i.e. what discourse strategies do the speakers use to allow for a smooth transition from one topic to the next?
- Who do you consider has 'control of the floor', e.g. who has the longest turns? Who determines the next speaker's turn?
- Now reflect on a situation in your clinical practice where you and another person (colleague or patient) are in conversation. Do you find that you finish each other's sentences? Why do you think that is? What does it tell you about your relationship and your understanding and approach to the clinical situation?

During our everyday conversations we often find ourselves in situations where we have to 'correct' what we have said, we 'search for the right word' or we feel we need to provide an explanation. Sometimes we might find ourselves saying something and almost before we have started to speak we change our mind about how we are going to formulate the utterance – a proposition, an answer or a question etc. Sometimes we overtly correct what we have said, or we reformulate what we have said, so intent are we to express the proposition clearly and ensure understanding on the part of our interlocutor – what CA regards as *troubles talk*. Such talk signals the collaborative nature of our conversation and our consideration for the other person and the relationship of the message to that person. *Troubles talk* is of concern to us as health professionals because it occurs not only in everyday conversations, but in health situations, as can be seen from the following two extracts of interactions between nurses and patients in health-assessment situations. The first illustration is an extract from the assessment of Mrs Y by Sara, a community nurse.

Illustration 2.6

Sara, a registered nurse, is assessing Mrs Y's health needs and asking about her social activities following her husband's death.

Sara:	... after you came back from overseas what did you do with yourself?
Mrs Y:	well after I came back I er (...) as a matter of fact
	after my husband died through him being with him continually all the
	time I found it very hard to get back into (...) the em (...) well
	(...)

In Illustration 2.6 we see that Mrs Y is 'correcting' herself as she offers an explanation to Sara for how difficult it is to re-establish her social life.

The Illustration 2.7 is an extract taken from Cheryth's assessment of Mrs S.

Illustration 2.7

165 Cheryth:	Has the doc have you mentioned to your doctor
166	the breathlessness?

Here we see Cheryth correcting herself, changing the agency from 'the doc' to 'you'

Conversation analysis is concerned with describing details of *conversational repair* and considers the collaborative style of the interlocutors as they manage what is generally regarded in CA as communicative 'trouble'. In interactions, unsatisfactory comprehension of the other person's turn, or, for that matter, an unacceptable response for whatever reason, is often indicated as an element which demands attention. We can signal this disturbance (or 'trouble') to perhaps what we expected to hear in a number of ways both verbally (by asking overt questions and/or use of intonation) or non-verbally, exemplified in the following table.

Example	Behaviour
Slight look of puzzlement	e.g. raising of the eyebrows
Minimal query	e.g. (i) 'Sorry?' (ii) 'Beg your pardon'
Questioning repeat (1)	i.e. an 'echo question' (one form of request for confirmation)
Questioning repeat (2) (with contrastive stress on repairable)	e.g. 'He consulted with Malcolm?' (rising tone)
Questioning paraphrase (often with 'so' and question tag - another form of request for confirmation	e.g. 'So your GP prescribed Erythromycin [paraphrase of information previously given by interlocutor] did she?' (tag question)
Questioning partial repeat (with	e.g. 'You prescribed antibiotics, steroids and ...?'

repairable portion left open)	(rising tone)
Explicit request for clarification (1)	e.g. 'What do you mean exactly?'; 'I'm sorry I don't understand, do you mean X?'
Explicit request for clarification (2) (proposing a specific replacement)	e.g. 'You mean … X?' (another form of request for confirmation)
Explicit request for clarification (3) proposing alternatives	e.g. 'Do you mean X … or Y?'
Explicit request for elaboration	e.g. 'Could you tell me more about what you mean by X?'

Similarly, there are a number of ways in which one can 'repair' the 'trouble'; for example, you might:

- slow down/repeat more clearly (particularly in a situation where your interlocutor has a sensory impairment or is a foreign language speaker, or where the interlocutor looks puzzled);
- paraphrase/reformulate what they have said as a check;
- make more explicit/contextualise/topicalise what the interlocutor has said;
- explicate or elaborate;
- code switch (for example where the interlocutor may be from another locality and speaking a different dialect; or a practitioner may switch from using medical to lay terminology to ensure patient understanding);
- make an overt appeal for assistance/give assistance, e.g. ask a direct question (or an indirect question in a situation where a direct question might cause embarrassment or loss of face).

Reflective learning 2.8: Repairs and clarification

Returning to the interaction between Cheryth and Mrs S in Interaction 2.2:

- What do you think are the indicators which suggest a need for clarification or repair of an utterance? How do you think clarification is given or a repair made; i.e. what discoursal strategies are deployed in doing this?
- Reflect on a conversation you have had with a friend. Identify utterances where either of you self-repaired/corrected an utterance.

2.3.6   Insertion sequences and side sequences

Schegloff (1972) states that typical of repair and clarification of 'moves' (and the move[s] in response) are insertions into the conversation, what conversation analysts have called 'insertion sequences' (Schegloff 1972) or 'side sequences' (Jefferson 1972). The effect of these sequences is to put the main dialogue temporarily 'on hold' until the 'trouble' is fixed – or repaired. The 'trouble' might be just a minor issue, but, whether minor or not, it must be repaired or clarified so that the conversation can continue without confusion. Examples of such insertions are seen in Illustration 2.8. If we now look at an extract of a transcript of conversation between a nurse and a patient in an aged care facility, we see how the patient (Mrs H) returns to her answer to Elaine's question (line 67).

Illustration 2.8

Elaine (nurse), assessing Mrs H's health status in an aged care facility

67 Elaine:	You're as independent as possible
68 Mrs H:	Oh yes they leave me to do things that I can do by myself
69 Elaine:	That's good
70 Mrs H:	They stand back and watch and just wait for me to say 'help' you know
71 Elaine:	That's good
72 Mrs H:	No they're very good.

Elaine listened to Mrs H explaining how her independence was encouraged, putting the assessment procedure 'on hold' as Mrs H attended to what conversation analysts would regard as troubles talk. In this instance Mrs H appears to believe that her response to Elaine's question in line 67 needed further explanation.

2.4   Summary

In exploring the contribution that CA makes to our understanding of how we use discourse to achieve our goals, the discussion in this chapter has examined the minutiae of interactions between nurses and patients at various sites of engagement, i.e. in assessment situations in healthcare facilities: the home, a rehabilitation unit and an aged care facility. Keeping close to the transcripts of data, you have engaged in activities which have allowed you to consider and analyse the means whereby interactions are managed.

Our proposition is that utterances can rarely be seen in isolation; always they are considered in apposition to one another. You have seen that discourse consists of turns between speakers that are not random but follow a pattern to which speakers subscribe. There is a structure in the resulting interaction made up of sequences of utterances – adjacency pairs where, for example, an offer is followed by an acceptance, a statement by an acknowledgement, a question by an answer and sometimes an extension of the response. You have seen too that sometimes the second or third part of a sequence is not technically 'adjacent' but appears later in the interaction. Of note also is that interlocutors repair and clarify their utterances, insert sequences, and by so doing ensure a shared understanding between the interlocutors, an essential attribute of healthcare discourse. All of this indicates the cooperative nature that makes for successful discourse, enabling the achievement of professional and discoursal goals.

Our exploration also indicated that rather than being 'messy', successful discourse is rule-governed. These rules do not always exist in the consciousness of the interlocutors, but are 'absorbed' by them through their exposure to interactions in the language community. This idea of an increasing 'discourse experience' raises the question of how persons who engage with the health community for the first time come to know what these 'rules' are, and how they contribute to the smooth running of the system of the healthcare institution, and what the unwritten rules are for what is permissible or impermissible in health discourse. For example, who actually is allowed to initiate turns in particular contexts, or 'hold the floor' with longer turns, or interrupt others? Who in fact holds power? While this learning by experience can be daunting for people who are native speakers and members of the local culture, for people who are members of different ethnic groups and do not share the cultural values, beliefs and behaviours of the local population, there is potential for considerable break-down in communication between patient and carer.

In considering the complexities of the discourse of interlocutors in the local situation and exploring the rule-governed nature and management of the inter-actions, you have also examined what the discourse resources are that are available to, and used by, interlocutors in their interactions. But you might also consider the World of Communication model (Chapter 1) and the factors which determine the discourse choices so that you can achieve your goals and contribute to the developing relationship of interlocutors in healthcare. The factors which govern our responses, actions and discourse include, for example, those of age, gender, education, occupation and above all the state of health and (different) understandings of the health situation by the interlocutors. One might argue that while CA is a useful tool, enabling us to discover the minutiae of utterances which allow us to co-construct our discourse (making for successful interactions), our discourse is produced against a backcloth of a complex social life. Our reading and reflections so far will underpin our study in subsequent chapters. Chapter 3 examines further the management of conversations and the use of available resources which contribute to the developing relationships within healthcare.

3   Common Purposes or Cross Purposes?

Concepts to be introduced, explored and applied

- Interactive frames and knowledge schemas
- Footing and participant roles
- Interpreter-mediated interactions
- Trust

Objectives of this chapter

After studying the issues addressed in the chapter, you will:

- understand the concept of *framing* as it applies to interactions, particularly in healthcare settings;
- use the concepts of framing and footing to describe some of the ways in which misunderstandings and miscommunication can occur in interactions between professional colleagues, as well as in interactions between clinicians and their clients/patients;
- appreciate some of the complexities involved in interpreter-mediated interactions in healthcare settings;
- become aware of different definitions of trust, and of some ways in which trust can be built through interactions.

3.1   Introduction

The main theoretical framework introduced here in this chapter is *interactive framing*. We can trace the notion of framing to Bateson (1955), who drew attention to the fact that participants must understand 'what is going on' at any given moment in an interaction in order to interpret the messages (verbal and non-verbal) of the other participants. A well-known example used by Bateson concerns the use of frames by animals to interpret identical actions as being part of 'playing' or 'fighting', and to respond accordingly. The sociologist Erving Goffman set out a comprehensive theory of framing in his book entitled *Frame Analysis* (Goffman 1974), using the question 'what is it that's going on here?' as his point of departure. The key principle to keep in mind is that our perspective on the particular frame in which a given activity is taking place will determine how we interpret utterances or actions of others.

In general, people are very skilled in 'knowing' what frame is being invoked at any given point in an interaction. This is because we all have expectations about the way in which people interact; some of these expectations are built up through experience interacting within a particular sociocultural environment, while others may be more related to our professional knowledge, relating to the way in which encounters proceed in our particular professional spheres.

To illustrate the insights that can come from an interactive framing approach, we will consider two interactions.

3.1.1   Discourse as a focus for discussion

Interaction 3.1

Anna (an occupational therapist), John (a speech pathologist) and Claire (a physiotherapist) work together at a rehabilitation hospital. They have come together in Anna's office for a short, informal meeting to co-ordinate their assessments of a few patients who have recently been transferred to their centre for an inpatient rehabilitation programme.

1 Anna:	OK, I'll just get a .. pen here, and then I can keep
2	track of what we //decide
3 John:	//good idea .. thanks
4 Anna:	Right, so who should we start with?
5 Claire:	Maybe Mr Nguyen? I was planning to see him this
6	afternoon so it'd be good to know when you both want
7	to ah (.) assess him
8 Anna:	OK great I'll put that down [writes] u::m I was hoping
9	to see him on Wednesday morning if that wouldn't ah
10	interfere with what you wanted to do, John?
11 John:	I've already seen him briefly ah (.) yesterday so I was
12	thinking of a full assessment early next week so–
13 Anna:	- next week did you say?
14 John:	ah (.) yeah (.) why? Do you think I should see him
15	sooner?
16 Anna:	no no no I mean for the notes

In the scenario above, Anna, John and Claire all bring their respective health professional roles to the meeting. As they all need to see Mr Nguyen in the next few days, the purpose of the meeting is to plan the timing of their assessments in a coordinated way. Anna, however, takes on an additional role, that of a note-taker. If we consider 'what is going on' in this interaction, we can identify two frames:

Frame 1: 'Schedule coordination'

Frame 2: 'Record keeping'

At first glance, the second frame may seem to be of very minor importance, but a correct interpretation of the intended meaning of Anna's utterance 'next week, did you say?' depends on the other participants' ability to perceive that a new frame (Frame 2 above) has been invoked. From the transcript, it appears that John believes that this utterance is made in the context of the 'schedule coordination' frame, and responds as though the wisdom of his plan is being questioned by Anna. Anna rapidly corrects his misinterpretation by clarifying that her question was in fact intended 'for the notes', which in effect makes explicit the fact that she is invoking a different frame.

Interaction 3.2

John (a speech pathologist) is carrying out a language assessment of Mr Nguyen, a 75-year-old man with aphasia following a stroke two weeks ago. Prior to the stroke, Mr Nguyen spoke Vietnamese fluently with his family and friends in the Vietnamese community, and also spoke limited English. John has therefore arranged an interpreter (Christine) to assist with the assessment of Mr Nguyen's language abilities following the stroke. As part of the standard assessment, John shows Mr Nguyen a picture and asks him to describe what he sees. (In this interaction, English translations of utterances in Vietnamese are placed in parentheses.)

1 John:	OK? so in this ah formal test (.) if I could get you to
2	(.) when you're translating back to me the responses (.)
3	to say word for word what he says (...) and also if
4	there's any incorrect pronunciation of the letters (.) if
5	you could just let me know =
6 Christine:	[nods] OK
7 John:	= about it as well (.) OK?
8	can you tell me what's happening in this picture?
9 Christine:	(Mr Nguyen, can you look at this picture)
10 Mr Nguyen:	(yes) [looks at picture]
11 Christine:	(you look at this picture, can you tell him what's in it?)

12 Mr Nguyen:	(here is a boy…boy…falling down…is it right?)
13 Christine:	um the boy is falling down
14 John:	[writes] - anything else?
15 Christine:	(and?)
16 Mr Nguyen:	(and this girl…she…she's catching …can't do it…can't
17	catch it)
18 Christine:	(catch what?)
19 Mr Nguyen:	(catch the biscuits)
20 Christine:	all right (.) the girl can't catch the biscuits
21 John:	[writes] - the girl can't catch the biscuits
22 Christine:	(and what? continue to talk)
23 Mr Nguyen:	(talk about this?)
24 Christine:	(you talk about it .. talk about whatever you see)
25 Christine:	he said 'talk about this?' and I said 'whatever you
26	see'
27 John:	OK
28 Mr Nguyen:	(what is this?) – [points to picture]
29 Christine:	I don't know what this is – [points to picture]
30 John:	is that what he said?
31 Christine:	yes
32 John:	looks to me like um like a hedge of u::m (.) a plant
33	hedge (.) or maybe some flowers
34 Christine:	(it's probably a hedge or some flowers)
35 John:	what do you think might happen when the mother
36	turns around?
37 Christine:	(when the mother turns around, what will she think?)
38 Mr Nguyen:	(mother turns around (.) must catch her son)
39 Christine:	If the mother turns around she must catch her son.
40 John:	OK, that's fine (…) can I just ask um in terms of his
41	speech production (.) are the sounds easy to
42	understand?
43 Christine:	[nods] - mm (.) mm
44 John:	are they (.) correct?
45 Christine:	mm (.) the sounds are correct – [nods]

Reflective learning 3.1: Roles and expectations

Consider Interaction 3.2 above and try to answer the following questions. We will work through this example later in this chapter, drawing on concepts introduced below in Section 3.2.

- What sorts of expectations do you think the interpreter and speech pathologist would have about the way in which this clinical encounter will unfold?
- How would they have formed these expectations (i.e. what would they be based upon)?
- Identify some instances in the interaction where the interpreter (Christine) appears to be performing what you would consider a 'normal' interpreter's role (i.e. interpreting from one language into another).
- Next, identify some points in the discourse where Christine appears to step out of this normative interpreting role; how would you characterise the role(s) that she adopts in these turns? (As we will see later, this is linked to the different frames that can be identified in the course of this interaction.)
- Why do you think that some of John's utterances are not interpreted into Vietnamese, and how does Christine 'decide' which utterances to interpret into the other language?
- Do your observations (in the reflective tasks above) tell you something about the different activities that are 'going on' in this scenario? Can you anticipate how these might relate to the various frames in operation here? (Hint: One way of defining the frames would be to look for sequences of turns where the interpreter is 'interpreting' the language tests as administered by the speech pathologist, as opposed to turns in which the speech pathologist is addressing the interpreter directly to seek further information.)

3.2   Interactive frames and knowledge schemas

Central to the concept of interactive framing is the way that expectations shape our understanding of events. In working out 'what it is that is going on here', we draw on past experience and knowledge to arrive at what seems to us to be the most likely interpretation of a given event or utterance. In Interaction 3.2, for instance, when Christine, says 'I don't know what this is' (line 29), John guesses (although he needs to confirm it) that this is likely to be an 'interpreted' utterance of Mr Nguyen's, rather than a statement by Christine about something that she cannot identify in the picture. At other points in the interaction, however, Christine does speak 'for herself' rather than interpreting (e.g. 'and I said "whatever you see"' – lines 25–26), so John must draw on his experience to decide what seems to be the most likely frame in which to understand the meaning of each utterance. This is for the most part a subconscious and automatic process. As Tannen (1993: 14) points out, it would not be possible to function in a life in which every experience was approached as a completely 'novel' occurrence, unrelated to anything that had gone before.

Like Goffman, Tannen and Wallat (1993) explain that interactive frames can be seen as defining 'what is going on' at any moment in an interaction, and stress that this information is vital in order for participants to know how to interpret any utterance, movement or gesture. They highlight the importance of individuals' expectations about people, objects, settings and events in the world, and they refer to these expectations as *knowledge schemas*. Their study is particularly relevant for our purposes, as it applies the concept of interactive framing to a clinical encounter. We therefore present this study in some detail here.

Tannen and Wallat analyse an interaction involving a paediatrician, mother, and child with cerebral palsy, focusing on the way in which one of the participants in their encounter (the paediatrician) juggles the competing frames which characterise this encounter. A major finding of their study is that the different knowledge schemas of the mother and the paediatrician (that is, the expectations that each has built up through past experiences of the world) tend to trigger frame shifts throughout the encounter. For instance, when discussing the child's recent general health, the mother expresses concern about her poor motor abilities and noisy breathing, which (for the mother) are part of a schema of 'poor health'. The doctor, who has seen many children with cerebral palsy, sees the child's motor abilities and noisy breathing as features that would be expected with cerebral palsy, and (for the doctor) they are thus not part of a schema of 'poor health' for this child.

Throughout the consultation, the paediatrician shifts between an 'examination' frame and a 'consultation' frame in an attempt to address both her own goals and the mother's goals for the encounter. In addition, the paediatrician is making a video for medical residents and at times reports to the camera as she conducts the physical examination. There is therefore a third 'teaching frame' in operation. As the interaction unfolds, the paediatrician can been seen to juggle the demands of the competing frames (answering the mother's questions, conducting the examination, keeping the child amused, and reporting to the recording camera). The authors conclude that the need to manage the conflicting demands of different frames can make the interaction burdensome for a doctor, and admire the skills of this particular doctor in managing these demands as effectively as she does.

In her study of interpreter-mediated interactions in a variety of contexts (including healthcare), Wadensjö (1998) also draws on the work of Erving Goffman in her analyses, particularly his concept of the *participation framework*. The basic idea behind the participation framework is that the organisation of spoken interaction ultimately results from participants' continuous evaluations and re-evaluations of speaker-hearer's roles, at the turn-by-turn level. Some participants are 'ratified' (i.e. have a legitimate role to participate at that point), while others are 'non-ratified' (including inadvertent overhearers and intentional eavesdroppers). The ratified participants can be further classified into those who are 'addressed' at a given point by the speaker and those who are present, and presumed to be listening, but who are not addressed directly at that moment. Non-addressed participants may become addressed participants if invited to speak, or if they take the initiative to enter the conversation and the other participants yield 'the floor' to them (see Chapter 2). For example, a father may attend a general practice consultation together with his teenage son, even though only the son is the patient for the purposes of that particular consultation. In such a situation, the father may be present but not actively participating during much of the consultation. However, the son may invite his father to participate at certain points by checking his own recollection of particular details. The doctor may also invite the father to participate by asking him if he has any particular questions. Finally, the father may jump in to the interaction at his own discretion if he wishes to contribute information or ask a question.

When exploring the ways in which people participate in interactions, it is useful to go deeper than a description of 'speakers' and 'hearers' (addressed or non-addressed). Goffman's concept of *production format* allows us to do this. In this model, an individual can act as *animator* (a mere mouthpiece giving sound to an utterance), *author* (responsible only for the assembly and synthesis of information and giving it form by composing/scripting the actual lines) or *principal* (assuming complete responsibility for the utterance and the intentions and beliefs which gave rise to it). It is thus possible for one to speak as animator only, as animator and author, or as animator, author and principal.

The important point here is that a person will listen differently to the utterances of others, depending on the way that they expect to respond (or participate) in the interaction. In other words, the way in which you attune yourself to the words of another person depends on the subsequent action that you expect (or are expected) to take with respect to what one hears. If listeners do not know in advance what they will be required to 'do' with the information that they receive, they will be unsure about the alignment that they take to the speaker's utterance. In short, they will not know 'how to listen' to what is being said. This is particularly pertinent to interpreters, as Wadensjö (1998) explains.

We have discussed the ways in which mismatches in knowledge schemas can bring about frame shifts in interactions, and have also considered the importance (for smooth communication) of a shared understanding (between participants) of the particular frame in operation at any given point. The concept of *footing* is closely associated with the notion of framing in discourse. Goffman (1981: 128) defines footing as 'the alignment we take up to ourselves and the others present as expressed in the way we manage the production or reception of an utterance'. We can expect, then, that participants will adopt a particular footing that is consistent with their understanding of the particular frame in operation at any point in an interaction. Concrete illustrations of exactly what constitutes 'footing' from an interactional perspective vary. Some writers use the term in a 'general' sense to describe different ways of dealing with and talking to other participants in an interaction, while others have tried to define the term more precisely. Levinson (1988), for instance, conceptualises footing as a 'participant role'. For our purposes, we will consider footing as the 'inner' moment-by-moment positioning of participants in an interaction, and the frame as the 'outer' level, describing what is going on in the interaction at a particular point.

In Interaction 3.1, for instance, where Anna says '<u>next </u>week, did you say?' (line 13), her footing with respect to John is one that involves 'checking and confirming', although John initially perceives Anna's footing at this moment to be one of 'questioning and challenging'. The footing that John adopts in his response to Anna will therefore depend on his interpretation of the footing that she has adopted in the preceding utterance addressed to him. Thus, in addition to the framing ambiguity at this point in the encounter (line 13), there is also a closely associated confusion with regard to interpretation of footings.

3.3   Frames and footings illustrated

To illustrate the concepts of interactive frames, knowledge schemas, footings and participant roles, we will now work through Interaction 3.2 in detail. You may also like to look back at your responses to the activities in Reflective learning 3.1. Detailed analysis of similar examples can be found in Roger and Code (forthcoming).

In order to identify the frames in operation in Interaction 3.2, it is useful to start by thinking about 'what is going on' in this interaction. The most obvious activity involves John assessing Mr Nguyen's aphasia by administering a set of language tests, assisted by the interpreter Christine. We could therefore identify a 'testing' frame. However, at some points in the interaction, John gives instructions to Christine (lines 1–7) or asks her questions about Mr Nguyen's performance (lines 40–45). No actual testing is occurring at these points, so we could identify a second frame here: a 'discussion' frame.

Line 7 marks a 'shift' from the initial discussion frame to the testing frame. Christine obviously recognizes that John's instructions are not part of the 'testing' frame, as she responds directly to what he says, rather than interpreting it for the client, Mr Nguyen. She also recognizes the shift back to the 'discussion' frame at line 40, as she once again responds to John's question, rather than interpreting it into Vietnamese. Subtle cues such as John's speaking volume and the ways that he directs his gaze, as well as the content of his utterances, serve to 'mark' these frame shifts. Christine therefore recognises where she is expected to respond as 'principal' to John's questions, and where she needs to assume the role of an 'animator' or 'author' by interpreting the test items in Vietnamese. Picking up these frame shifts is crucial, because the frame in operation determines the way in which Christine needs to respond, and therefore determines the way in which she listens to what John is saying (and vice versa).

Communication becomes more difficult when participants have to 'manage' the demands of several frames at once, as illustrated in Tannen and Wallat's study (1993). All participants in an interaction need to be able to perceive the frame in operation at a given moment in order to respond appropriately. At lines 29–30 in Interaction 3.2, however, we see a momentary ambiguity in framing. Following an utterance from Mr Nguyen, Christina says (in English), 'I don't know what this is'. It appears that John is uncertain for a moment whether Christine is speaking as an animator/author (i.e. interpreting Mr Nguyen's words) or as a principal (i.e. letting John know that *she* does not recognise something in the picture). John therefore asks, 'Is that what he said?' (line 30) in order to clarify the frame in operation, before responding to the actual question.

Why do frame shifts occur in this encounter? In the study by Tannen and Wallat (1993) discussed above, we saw that *mismatches in the knowledge schemas* of the participants was an important factor in triggering shifts in frames. This is also true of the interaction between Mr Nguyen, Christine and John. As a Vietnamese–English interpreter, Christine obviously has a much more comprehensive knowledge schema for the Vietnamese language than has John. As a speech pathologist, John has a highly developed knowledge schema for aphasia which is probably not shared by Christine. Shifts in and out of the 'discussion' frame are necessary (1) for John to brief Christine on what he needs to know in assessing people with aphasia and (2) for John to access Christine's impressions of Mr Nguyen's Vietnamese, a language that he (John) does not speak. The second of these two points raises a controversial issue for the interpreting profession, as the interpreter is being asked to provide information that falls well outside the interpreting function. Such issues are outside the scope of the discussion in this chapter, but are considered in detail in Roger and Code (2011).

How are frame shifts in interactions initiated, or triggered? In an analysis of interactions in a medical audiology clinic, Coupland and Jaworski (1997) show how changes in footing can trigger shifts in frames; that is, a change in the alignment that one participant takes up to another can signal that a change is taking place in terms of 'what is going on' at that moment in the interaction. As we have seen in Interaction 3.1, Anna's shift in footing towards John triggers a frame shift, but this cue is initially missed by John, leading to momentary confusion about why she might be challenging his decision. In this instance, the ambiguity is rapidly resolved, but in some cases participants may continue to operate in different frames for extended periods. An example would be a counselling session in which the client believes that a counsellor is 'telling him what he should do', while the counsellor believes that he is 'helping the client to see his options'. If the mismatch becomes evident during the course of the consultation, the counsellor may opt to *reframe* the encounter overtly.

Reflective learning 3.2: Interactive framing

Consider an encounter that you have had with a colleague (from the same profession or another profession) or a consultation with a patient/client where you felt that the communication did not seem to proceed smoothly.

- What frames can you identify in this interaction?
- What sorts of mismatches in knowledge schemas (if any) were evident relating to some of the topics under discussion?
- Did you and the other person seem to share an understanding of 'what was going on' at various points in the encounter?
- Do the concepts discussed so far in this chapter help to explain why the communication seemed less than optimal?

3.4   Trust

In the discussion in this chapter so far, we have explored the importance of an individual's *expectations* (based on previous experiences) in determining how they interpret the actions and words of others from a framing standpoint. Expectations and experiences also underpin another key concept that we can examine from a discourse perspective: *trust*.

Issues of trust are of course central to relationships between healthcare practitioners and their patients, as well as the inter-professional relationships between the practitioners. What do we mean by trust? Dunleavy, Chory and Goodboy point out that trust is 'developed based on a prior relational history with the individual and includes expectations about the individual's behavior' (2010: 244). These expectations concern the likelihood that an individual will exhibit what could be called 'trustworthy behaviors' which include:

- telling the truth,
- communicating accurately and openly,
- behaving predictably,
- not hurting others.

Maguire, Phillips and Hardy (2001) comment that *predictability* (one of the 'trustworthy behaviors' listed above) is the common element that runs through many of the different approaches to defining the concept of trust. Put simply, if we can confidently predict what another person will do in a given situation, we will trust them. However, you may have recognised instantly that such a definition of trust seems rather hollow, in that it does not embody any concern for the wellbeing of the other person. This missing element is what Maguire et al. (2001) refer to as *goodwill*. 'Weak' forms of trust, they argue, are based solely on predictability, while 'stronger' forms of trust also embody an element of goodwill. On this basis, they present (building on the work of others) three forms of trust. The first two of these embody only the element of predictability:

Calculus-based trust: This weak form of trust exists when a 'trustor' can predict what another person will do in a given situation, *and* is able to control the other person's behaviour through a system of rewards and punishments.

Knowledge-based trust: This weak form of trust exists when a trustor has sufficient knowledge of a person to be able to predict what that person will do in a given situation, even though the trustor does not have (or does not seek) control over the other person's behaviour.

Reflective learning 3.3: Concepts of trust

Before we consider the 'stronger' form of trust described by Maguire et al. (2001), consider the calculus-based and knowledge-based forms above.

- Do they represent (in any way) the concept of 'trust' as you understand it, or do they seem to describe something quite different from your understanding of what 'trust' is?
- Do these particular forms of trust sometimes form the basis of professional-client relationships in healthcare?
- Do these particular forms of trust sometimes describe relationships between healthcare professionals, or between those in various roles in institutions such as hospitals?

We would argue that such definitions of trust are, for the most part, incomplete characterisations of the concept of trust from the perspective of most healthcare practitioners. Indeed, some people may reject them altogether as characterisations of trust. When we consider the notion of power in Chapter 11, you may like to reflect back on knowledge-based and calculus-based trust, and consider the parallels that exist. We will turn now to the third form of trust that Maguire et al. (2010) identify:

> *Identification-based trust:* This is a strong form of trust, in that the trustee identifies with (or at least acknowledges and respects) the other person's needs, values and choices.

There is thus an element of goodwill in this form of trust that is conspicuously absent in the weaker forms of trust described above. The trustor, in turn, recognises the goodwill and over time becomes confident that this goodwill is a stable and predictable part of the relationship. Candlin (2010) points out that trust is best viewed as a *process* rather than a state. Identification-based trust, with its embodiment of goodwill, opens up the possibility for trust to be 'built' or 'earned' as part of a process. Goodwill must of course be demonstrated through words or actions if it is to lead to a trusting relationship, and here we can see that trust can be seen as something that *develops through interactions* (or we might say *discourse*) over a period of time.

3.4.1   Discourse as a focus for discussion

Interaction 3.3 (data from Roger and Code 2011)

Susan (a speech pathologist) and Iska (an interpreter) are carrying out a language assessment of a bilingual Tagalog-English speaker (Pedro) with aphasia. This is the first time that Iska and Susan have worked together, and they have not previously met each other.

1 Susan:	OK, I'm going to ask you some questions now (.) what
2	do you write with?
3 Iska:	may ilan ho akong itatanong sa inyo (..) anong ginagamit
4	ninyo pag nagsusulat kayo?
5 Pedro:	my name
6 Susan:	OK, I'll say it again (.) what do you write with?
7 Iska:	sasabihin ko ho uli ang tanong (..) pag ho nagsusulat,
8	ano ho ang ginagamit ninyo para kayo makapag sulat?
9 Pedro:	ballpen
10 Susan:	mm(..) did you change the phrasing then?
11 Iska:	ye::s
12 Susan:	how did you word it?
13 Iska:	I (.) I just told him 'whenever you write, what do you
14	use to be able to write?'
15 Susan:	OK

Reflective learning 3.4: More on trust

Looking at the encounter above, consider the professional relationship between Susan and Iska.

- How do issues of trust arise in this particular event (a language assessment conducted with the assistance of an interpreter)?
- Are there any points at which one participant seems not to trust the other? How is this evident from the interaction?
- Are there any points at which one participant seems to feel that she does not have the trust of the other? How is this evident from the discourse?

In Interaction 3.3, the speech pathologist (Susan) is not a Tagalog speaker, and she is thus reliant on the interpreter (Iska) in this regard. Ideally she would probably like to reach a point where she feels that Iska's interpreting is *accurate and complete* (see the 'trustworthy behaviors' in our earlier discussion) and that her approach to interpreting in this setting is both *predictable* and underpinned by *goodwill*. As they have not previously worked together, however, the process of developing trust at this point (approximately 15 minutes into the assessment) is at a very early stage.

In line 10, Susan initiates a frame shift, interrupting the 'testing' frame to address Iska directly. While her question ('Did you change the phrasing then?') could be a simple inquiry, it could also be taken as a 'pre-criticism', as aphasia test items are generally repeated verbatim if a repetition is necessary. Iska is probably unaware of this, being accustomed (as an interpreter) to facilitating communication by paraphrasing utterances that have not been understood the first time. Her hesitant delivery in line 11 (ye::s) suggests that she may be concerned that she has inadvertently 'done something wrong', and that this may impede the building of a trusting relationship between the two professionals.

In this instance, we can identify Susan's frame shift in line 10, and Iska's hesitation in line 11 as significant interactional features that have a bearing on the building of trust. Once again, we must bear in mind that trust is part of a process, and what can be gleaned from a short extract such as Interaction 3.3 is very limited. However, if (hypothetically speaking) Susan were to initiate similar frames shifts throughout the encounter, it would be possible that the cumulative effect of such 'questioning' moves might lead Iska to feel quite clearly that Susan does not trust her.

It is interesting that as this particular encounter unfolds, Iska asks Susan on another occasion whether it would be all right for her to rephrase a particular item. By doing this, she is demonstrating 'predictable' behaviour as well as showing goodwill in respecting Susan's indirectly expressed wish to be made aware of any rephrasing that Iska does. This is likely to foster the building of trust between the two professionals.

The example above is just one illustration of the ways in which we can look for particular discourse features that are important in the building of trusting relationships. In professional–patient encounters, both O'Grady (2011a) and Candlin and Crichton (2013) point out that trust is often built through empathy and rapport (see specifically the discussion by O'Grady and Candlin, 2013). Empathy is considered in detail in the following chapter, and you may (at that point) like to reflect on the links between 'empathy' and 'trust' as they are displayed through actual interactions.

3.5   Summary

From what we have seen in this chapter, both knowledge and expectations play a key role in communication in healthcare settings. Framing such knowledge and expectations turns out to be very relevant when we are exploring interactions between members of a team who have worked together for a long time (as in Interaction 3.1) or professionals (and/or professionals and clients) who are working together for the first time (as in Interaction 3.2). Footing provides a means of describing the particular alignment (in the sense of a position or stance) adopted by one participant at any given moment with respect to the other participants.

Trust is another concept that is grounded in expectations about another person's behaviour, and we have considered here just one example of the way in which trust is built up or eroded through interactional choices of participants. Throughout this book, you will encounter further examples of ways in which trust is built through interactions between healthcare professionals, and between clinicians and their clients.

Chapter 4 will provide additional perspectives on the positions or alignments that participants adopt in communicative encounters, with reference to the important associated concept of *face*.

4   Respecting Feelings and Perspectives

Concepts to be introduced, explored and applied

- Empathy and sympathy
- Affiliation
- Issues of face: threatening face, maintaining face, saving face

Objectives of this chapter
After completing the study of this chapter you will be able to:

- analyse the concepts of affiliation, empathy and sympathy;
- identify the variables associated with facework;
- appreciate the sensitive nature of facework;
- understand how such sensitivity affects interactions.

4.1   Introduction

We often hear how important it is for healthcare professionals to have *empathy* in dealing with their patients or clients, but exactly what 'empathy' is and how it is displayed (or not displayed) in healthcare consultations is less often discussed. In order to explore the notion of empathy in health communication, however, it is perhaps useful to begin with a working definition of the concept.

One of many ways of characterising empathy is provided by Halpern, who writes: 'In empathy one grasps, more or less, how the other person experiences her situation: at the same time the empathizer herself experiences the other's attitudes as presences, rather than as possibilities' (1996: 167). This view of empathy thus involves both understanding and a degree of emotional engagement with the other person; it is, in effect, a demonstration of *affiliation* with another person on a human level. Empathy can be distinguished from 'sympathy', which generally implies feelings of compassion for the plight or situation of another person. For this reason, 'empathy' (rather than sympathy) tends to be seen as a key humanistic element in healthcare encounters, although it must be acknowledged that the terms are often used interchangeably in lay conversation.

In this chapter, we will be concerned with what Ruusuvuori (2005) calls 'empathy in action'; that is, we will focus on ways in which empathy is (or is not) *displayed* through the participants' actual behaviour (both verbal and non-verbal). The other key concept explored in this chapter is that of *face*. Like empathy, 'face' is a term that is often used in everyday English, particularly as part of the phrases 'losing face' and 'saving face'. In order to understand how a person can lose face or save face when interacting with others, linguists have proposed systems for understanding the notion of face. We will explore one such system in this chapter, through the scenarios, commentary and activities that follow.

4.1.1   Discourse as a focus for discussion

Interaction 4.1

Interns Melanie and Kevin are friends as well as fellow interns at a large teaching hospital. They are required to work some overnight (on call) shifts as part of their internship, and Melanie has just completed one such shift.

1 Melanie:	That was the (.) ah busiest overnight shift I've ever had (..)
2	it just didn't stop from six o'clock til about half an hour ago=
3 Kevin:	[smiling] =no sleep then?
4 Melanie:	No way! I was flat out and um at one point John had to help
5	me out 'cos I just physically couldn't get down to emergency
6	and they'd called me three tim//es
7 Kevin:	//oh no (.) they really need um another
8	person to cover the new admissions through emerg//?ency//
9 Melanie:	// yes exa//ctly (.) I mean
10	I wanted to go down there but with so many sick people on the ward (.)
11	I mean what can you do?
12 Kevin:	Mm (.) I had the same problem last Sunday and when I finally
13	got to emergency they were not impressed as they'd been=
14 Melanie:	mm (.) mm [nods]
15 Kevin:	=calling me
16	for the past two hours...

Interaction 4.2

Maxine, an occupational therapist, is making a post-discharge home visit to Mrs Peterson, an 86-year-old woman who lives alone. Mrs Peterson left hospital about a week earlier, following a total hip replacement and a period of inpatient rehabilitation. Prior to discharge, Maxine had recommended (and offered to arrange) some minor bathroom modifications, but Mrs Peterson wanted to give the matter more consideration before proceeding.

1 Maxine:	you've been home a week now, I think?
2 Mrs P:	yes (.) six days actually that's right it is (.) six days (..)
3 Maxine:	that's right it is (.) six days (..) and how's it all been going (.) I mean
4	are you managing OK with all the things and how's it all been going
5	(.) I mean are you managing OK with all the things you need to do?
6 Mrs P:	yes well it was all going well until (.) ah yesterday morning when I
7	slipped in the shower and knocked my leg here you can see=
8 Maxine:	=oh no you
9	poor thing
10 Mrs P:	well it's not really as bad as it looks but it was pretty sore yesterday
11 Maxine:	mm (.) I'm sure it was (.) it's made a nasty bruise just – um, it
12	looks like you bumped it on the side of the tub (.) were you
13	you ah getting out of the shower when it happened?
14 Mrs P:	that's right (.) just got my feet in the wrong position and –
15	(.) here's me thinking how well I'm doing and then this
16	happens and (.) well it just knocks my confidence and makes
17	me feel (.) well, down, you know? (looks a little tearful)
18 Maxine:	(nods) sometimes that's a lot worse than a sore bruised leg isn't it?
19 Mrs P:	mm (.) exactly
20 Maxine:	well um feeling confident is really important and you know I
21	ah (.) I do think that um a hand rail in the shower and the
22	kinds of small modifications we were talking about last week
23	would really help a lot (.) ah with that (..) um confidence (.)
24	have you given it any more thought?

Reflective learning 4.1: Applying theory to practice

- What are some of the different ways (verbal and non-verbal) that one person can display empathy with another? What examples can you identify in Interactions 4.1 and 4.2?
- What sorts of strategies do people commonly use to display empathy in casual conversations between friends or colleagues (e.g. Interaction 4.1)?

(cont.)

Reflective learning 4.1 (cont.)

- How do health professionals display empathy in consultations with their patients or clients? How is it done in your profession?
- What obvious differences between the ways that empathy is displayed in Interaction 4.2 (a professional encounter) as compared with Interaction 4.1 (a personal encounter)? How might we account for these differences?

4.2   Empathy: What is it and how is it conveyed?

The word 'empathy' came into the English language in the early twentieth century as a translation of the German term *Einfühlung*. One of its early usages in psychology was to describe the process by which one person comes to 'know' another (Davis 1994). Since this time, many conceptualisations of empathy have been proposed by theorists, and the term has acquired various meanings as a 'lay' term as well. This may explain why healthcare professionals sometimes have differing understandings of exactly what empathy means, and what it involves.

Some theorists have defined empathy in purely affective terms, while others see empathy as having more cognitive dimensions. In healthcare practice, what we commonly refer to as 'empathy' clearly involves more than an 'emotional reaction' on the part of the practitioner; an 'understanding' is also necessary. Baron-Cohen (2003) sees empathy as 'tuning in' to another person's thoughts and feelings. He identifies a cognitive component which involves 'understanding the other's feelings and the ability to take their perspective' and an affective component, which is an appropriate emotional response to the other person's emotional state. It is important to remember that empathy is an 'attitude' that is reflected in the way that one person approaches an interaction with another.

We are focusing in this chapter on the ways in which empathy is displayed in discourse, which is important as it concerns the way in which a clinician conveys empathy to a client (or to a colleague, depending on the nature and the purpose of the interaction). Ruusuvuori (2005: 206) uses the term 'empathy in action' to describe the 'ways of conduct' that signal displays of empathy in clinical interactions. However, attempts at displaying empathy when in fact the clinician is not attending to the task of trying to understand the patient's feelings are often obvious in their deficiency, as we will discuss later.

For our purposes, therefore, it is useful to consider exactly how we recognise another person as empathic. Empathy is evident where an interlocutor acknowledges – verbally or non-verbally – the thoughts or feelings of another person.

The ways in which empathy is displayed will naturally vary according to the context of the encounter, the relationship between the people involved, the broader cultural context and individual personalities. Some common 'carriers' of empathy can, however, be identified – these are summarised in Table 4.1.

Table 4.1 Carriers of empathy

Non-verbal carriers of empathy	Considerations
Proxemics	This refers to the way in which participants are positioned in relation to each other. An arrangement where both speakers are at approximately equal eye levels at a physical distance that is appropriate to the cultural and interactional context is likely to be most conducive to displays of empathy.
Close and active listening	Showing a willingness to listen closely and carefully is essential, as empathy involves achieving a level of understanding of another person's thoughts and feelings. If someone feels that the other person has not paid sufficient attention to what they have said, they are not likely to believe that they have been understood. In many cultures, close listening involves maintaining an appropriate degree of eye contact, nodding, facial expression and the use of back channelling cues ('mm hm', 'yes', 'right', 'I see'). These markers of active listening are not universal however, as we will discuss further in Chapter 6.
Tone of voice and speech rate	A neutral tone of voice is probably most effective, and adopting an artificially 'soothing' or soft tone of voice is not likely to enhance one's ability to display empathy. A tone that is brusque, impatient, hurried, irritated or 'preachy' is unlikely to convey a sense of empathy.
Touch	Various degrees of physical contact are often a powerful part of displays of empathy. In the case of family or friends, this may involve putting an arm around the other person, or hugging them. In clinical or collegial interactions, touch (if it is used at all) is likely to be much more limited (e.g. briefly touching a person's arm or holding their hand). Individuals vary greatly in the degree to which they are comfortable touching others or being touched, and individual, cultural and institutional considerations sometimes mean that it is safer to avoid physical touch, particularly in professional encounters.

Acknowledgement through paraphrase	Empathy can be displayed by restating or paraphrasing salient elements of what the other person has said. This displays one participant's understanding of what the other has said, and allows the original speaker to confirm or correct it at the next turn. In a therapeutic relationship, it is important to ensure that paraphrasing is not done in a 'patronising' manner (Candlin 2008) that might make the other person feel as though they are being 'told' how they feel.
Statement of understanding	This refers to a short statement intended to signal understanding of the thoughts, feelings or experiences that the person is reporting.
Legitimising	Empathy can be displayed through comments or 'extensions' of a statement or commentary extension of speaker's utterance by another speaker, with the intention of validating or legitimising the sentiments, concerns or feelings that have been expressed.
'Pursuit' of the topic	A powerful way of displaying empathy is to 'pick up' on the thoughts or through further feelings expressed by the other person, and explore them further through questioning, commentary and/or discussion. The way in which this is done varies according to the 'purpose' of the encounter, and whether its goals are primarily social or professional. This is explored in detail in the discussion that follows

Reflective learning 4.2: Factors affecting displays of empathy

Look again at Interactions 4.1 and 4.2 and imagine the 'non-verbal' elements of communication that are not reflected in the transcript.

- How would these be optimised to display appropriate empathy?
- How might the gender and the cultural background of the participants affect the ways in which empathy was displayed in these scenarios? For instance, would Interaction 4.1 play out differently if 'Melanie' and 'Kevin' were both men, or both women? Similarly, how might Interaction 4.2 be different if both the occupational therapist and patient were men, rather than women (see Chapter 1 - The World of Communication)? We will consider these sorts of issues further in Chapter 6.
- Which of the verbal 'carriers' of empathy in Table 4.1 are exemplified in Interactions 4.1 and 4.2?
- What can you add to the list of 'carriers' of empathy outlined in Table 4.1?

4.3   Empathy in context

In conversations with family, friends or work colleagues, one of the common ways in which we display empathy with another person is to tell what Sacks (1992) refers to as a *second story*, in which we respond by talking about a similar problem or situation that we have experienced directly or through a third person. This is what Kevin does in his conversation with Melanie in Interaction 4.2 above; in his 'second story' he discloses similar problems in coping with the competing demands of the overnight shift, and in effect lets Melanie know that she is not alone in experiencing such difficulties, and not out of step in experiencing stress as a result.

In professional–client encounters, however, Ruusuvuori (2005) points out that the 'institutional task' generally demands that both parties work toward a solution to the problems that the client is experiencing. While telling a 'second story' may be a powerful way of demonstrating empathy, it does not necessarily move the interaction towards a solution to the problem. Indeed, there is a danger that the professional's own experience can upstage the patient, as in the case of a patient who told a palliative care nurse, 'We had a doctor here this morning. By the time we'd heard about his carcinoma, he hadn't much time for me …' (Hunt 1991: 936).

Telling a 'second story' also involves a level of self-disclosure that some clinicians (and patients) would see as out of keeping with the nature of the professional relationship. While the use of 'second stories' in healthcare consultations may be less common, there are situations when they may be used effectively. For instance, where one doctor consults a medical friend or colleague about her own health concerns, the 'treating' doctor may feel more at liberty to demonstrate empathy through self-disclosure, realising that the person seeking help will feel reassured to hear first-hand that another doctor has also experienced similar concerns.

Reflective learning 4.3: Second stories

- Can you think of any instances when you have used 'second stories' as a way of demonstrating understanding or empathy with a patient? What was the outcome?
- How common do you think the use of 'second stories' might be among members of your particular profession?
- Can you recall observing expressions of empathy (towards patients of colleagues) that struck you as particularly effective and appropriate to the context? How was empathy displayed in these instances?

Interaction 4.2 demonstrates ways in which a health professional displays empathy that also assist in meeting the needs of the 'institutional' task at hand. In line 10, Mrs Peterson comments that 'it's not as bad as it looks …', making reference to the obvious bruise on her leg. After *acknowledging* Mrs Peterson's experience of pain, Maxine picks up on the visible appearance of the bruised leg to seek more information about how the accident happened. Her displays of empathy thus lead smoothly into questions that elicit clinically useful information from Mrs Peterson. In line 18, Maxine expresses empathy by offering a *commentary* on Mrs Peterson's disclosure regarding her loss of confidence and despondent mood, which Mrs Peterson subsequently confirms as an accurate assessment. This allows Maxine to take up the issue of confidence (which Mrs Peterson has raised) to reintroduce the topic of home modifications as a possible solution. Thus, displays of empathy in this scenario tend to be followed by moves that address the institutional tasks of information-gathering and problem-solving, rather than being unconnected with the goals of the encounter.

The way in which empathy is woven into the consultation, rather than being expressed in a way that is divorced from the purpose of the encounter, is indicative of a degree of *professional communicative expertise* (see Chapter 10) on the part of the occupational therapist (OT) Maxine. Introducing the topic of home modifications (which Mrs Peterson has previously declined) is potentially sensitive and, by making the link with the issue of confidence, Maxine is able to raise the subject in a neutral manner, as the relevance to the previous turns is overtly established. Without this link, bringing up the topic of home modifications may have come across as being heavy handed on the part of the OT.

The importance of displaying empathy is often stressed in training or clinical examination settings for health professionals, where they may be assessed in part on their capacity to 'show empathy' when talking to patients. A possible pitfall is for the trainee to focus too much on the superficial displays of empathy, rather than seeing such displays as integral to their professional work. This can result in rather clumsy interactions, as illustrated in Interaction 4.3 from a clinical examination in which Cameron (a medical student) is taking a history from Ms Ellis, a 'patient' in a mock consultation.

Interaction 4.3

Cameron (a medical student) is taking a history from Ms Ellis, a 'patient' in a mock consultation.

1 Cameron:	Are you taking any medications at the moment?
2 Ms Ellis:	only aspirin ah (.) one in the morning (..) I was on aten- ah
3	atenolol for a while, but I got so::: dizzy with that you know, and
4	last Friday morning I passed out in the bathroom and gave my
5	husband a terrible fright
6 Cameron:	Really? I'm sorry to hear that. Um (.) do you smoke?

Although Cameron has gone through the motions of displaying empathy, the sudden topic shift that follows may make Ms Ellis (and indeed the examiners) wonder if Cameron's words really reflected an empathic attitude or whether he was merely trying to 'tick the empathy box'. His response is in fact closer to an expression of *sympathy* than of empathy, and the fact that it is not incorporated more seamlessly into the history-taking sequence may reflect (at least in part) Cameron's novice status. This illustrates that when we look for evidence of empathy in discourse, it is important to look beyond isolated phrases such as 'mm hm' or 'how terrible!' or 'I'm sorry to hear that', and consider the trajectory of the interaction as a whole. As we have discussed above, empathy is not an attitude to be adopted and displayed briefly and transiently, but is central to the business of attending to the professional task at hand.

Our discussion of Interactions 4.1, 4.2 and 4.3 has emphasised the value of looking at empathy in the context of the overall interaction, and not as something that can simply be 'inserted' at particular junctures. Pounds (2011) and O'Grady (2011b) note that empathy is sometimes taught (in clinical communication courses) with the aid of lists of useful phrases that the trainee can use to express empathetic sentiments. However, as both of these writers point out, reliance on such collections of 'stock phrases' risks oversimplifying the complex and important role that empathy plays in a consultation.

O'Grady (2011b) emphasises that empathy can be seen as a cooperative activity that is jointly achieved (or not achieved) by patient and clinician. In line with Ruusuvuori (2005), O'Grady points out that 'clinically effective empathy' is not simply a matter of showing that one has perceived, appreciated and understood a patient's feelings, but that 'empathy has clinical work to do' (2011b: 50). Taking a discourse analytic approach, she identified 'critical moments' (C.N. Candlin 1997) in general practice consultations where skilful displays of empathy on the part of the doctor have the capacity to 'turn' the consultation in ways that allow sensitive topics to be broached, with the emergence of potentially valuable clinical information. Missing such critical moments, by contrast, can close off opportunities for issues and information of clinical significance to be raised. O'Grady (2011b) provides a powerful illustration of this, through an example where a patient begins to disclose 'panic attack' symptoms in a tentative, embarrassed and almost apologetic manner, as if ready to retreat altogether from the topic at any moment. Through a skilful combination of gaze, body positioning, silence and verbal expressions of empathy and openness, the doctor is able to bring the consultation to a point where the issue is brought into the open 'as a matter that can be interpersonally but professionally discussed' (p. 50). Thus, while it is of course desirable that patients feel understood and accepted by their healthcare professionals, it is important to recognise that empathy also has a vital role in optimising the quality of clinical practice and care.

Reflective learning 4.4: Considering the other person in practice

In Interaction 4.1, Melanie admits that she was at times facing difficulties coping with her work overnight.

- How do you think Melanie felt about herself after the conversation, and about Kevin's impression of her as a 'competent person'? What evidence for your answers can you find in the actual interaction?
- From her words, who is Maxine (Interaction 4.2) suggesting needs to make the decision about such modifications? What 'common goal' (shared by Mrs Peterson and Maxine) does she use to try to persuade Mrs Peterson that this course of action would be a good idea?

4.4   Face and facework

As we discussed in Chapter 1, the simplest models of communication sometimes talk in terms of a message being 'sent' by one person and the same message being 'received' by another. However, we know from experience that the message that one person intends to send is not always the same message that the listener receives. We also know that in some cases ('small talk' for example) the actual information that is being exchanged is unimportant or redundant, but this does not stop people from exchanging it anyway. One of the factors that helps to explain these apparent paradoxes is the fact that communication is as much about shaping our relationships with others as it is about exchanging facts and opinions. What we say, and the way in which we say it, can serve to build, strengthen, strain or destroy our relationships with others, as it affects the self-images of those who are interacting with us, as well as determining the self-image that we project to others. This self-image is what we call *face*, and the elements of communication that are directed (consciously or unconsciously) at the self-images of ourselves and others are known as *facework*.

Brown and Levinson discuss the concept of face, defining it as:

The public self-image that every member wants to claim for himself, consisting of two related aspects: (a) negative face: the basic claim to territories, personal preserves, rights to non-distraction i.e. to freedom of action and freedom from imposition [and]

(b) positive face: the positive consistent self-image or 'personality' (crucially including the desire that this self-image be appreciated and approved of) claimed by interactants (Brown and Levinson 1987: 61).

They conceptualise face as wants, so that *negative face* becomes the want of individuals that their actions not be impeded by others, and *positive face* becomes the want of individuals that their actions/choices be desirable to at least some others. In any action where face is threatened, then, a positive politeness strategy is a form of redress directed to the addressee's positive face (i.e. making the person feel good), whereas a negative politeness strategy is directed to the addressee's negative face (i.e. reducing the apparent imposition). Note that the term *politeness* is being used in a particular sense here to refer to the maintenance of face (and *not* to class-conscious socially correct behaviour, which is another meaning sometimes associated with the word 'politeness').

In this framework, a strategy such as 'indirectness' would be classified as a negative politeness strategy because it is directed at the addressee's negative face, i.e. it respects this individual's presumed desire for freedom from imposition. By contrast, a strategy such as 'showing interest' is a positive politeness strategy, as it is directed at the addressee's desire to be liked or approved of by others.

In Brown and Levinson's framework, it is assumed that the content and boundaries inherent in the concept of face will vary from one culture to another, but that the social need to be aware of and orient oneself towards the face wants of others is universal. The universality of Brown and Levinson's framework is a matter of some controversy, but the framework itself is a useful starting point (although certainly not the only one) for looking at the way in which face can be threatened in professional–client and colleague–colleague interactions, and the way in which these potential or actual face threats can be mitigated.

In a similar vein, R. Lakoff (1973) proposed three 'rules of rapport' in interactions: (1) don't impose, (2) give options, and (3) make the receiver feel good. We can see that the first two rules are directed at the recipient's 'negative face', while the third rule is directed at the recipient's 'positive face'. These are (of course) not 'codified' rules, but tacit assumptions that underlie our ideas of polite and reasonable interactions. Naturally, they need to be interpreted in light of the context in which the interaction is taking place. In workplace contexts, for example, it is often expected that a 'boss' (manager, director, supervisor, etc.) will direct others to do something (breaking the first rule) and will not present a series of choices (breaking the second rule) when doing so. However, the way in which this 'directive' is performed – including the words that are used – will have the effect of either mitigating or intensifying the potential face threat. We will examine this specific issue in Chapter 5. First, however, we will consider the ways in which Interactions 4.1 and 4.2 illustrate various positive and negative politeness strategies.

In Interaction 4.1, Melanie tells Kevin about her busy overnight shift. In doing so, she discloses that she was unable to respond in a timely way to calls from the emergency department, and that she needed a colleague to help her out with the busy work. This is a potentially face-threatening disclosure, as Melanie's self-image as a competent intern is at stake. Kevin's responses are addressed at Melanie's *positive* face (making her feel 'approved of'), first by stating that the system (not Melanie) is at fault (lines 7–8) and then by recounting a similar situation that he faced and had difficulty managing (lines 12–13). The fact that Kevin and Melanie are both interns who do similar kinds of work, together with their friendship, makes it easier for them to empathise with each other, and the 'positive' face-saving strategies that Kevin uses arise quite naturally. By contrast, if Kevin had responded critically, by saying (for instance) 'you need to learn to prioritise your work', this would probably have intensified (rather than mitigated) the threat to Melanie's positive face, and she may have left the encounter feeling less than good about herself (and Kevin).

In Interaction 4.2, Maxine (the occupational therapist) clearly feels that Mrs Peterson would benefit from some modifications to her bathroom to make it safer for her to manage at home by herself. She uses politeness strategies directed at saving Mrs Peterson's face, but in this case they are directed at her *negative* face (i.e. a person's desire to make decisions for themselves and not be imposed upon). Maxine does not say, 'Look, you really must have handrails installed', but instead explains why she thinks Mrs Peterson would feel more confident with handrails and says, 'Have you given it any more thought?' (line 24). In addition to this indirect approach, it is also evident that Maxine's speech becomes rather tentative and hedged at this point, something we will explore in detail in Chapter 5. Using these so-called 'negative politeness strategies' (i.e. directed at the listener's negative face) in this sort of situation is in line with the fact that (1) it is Mrs Peterson's house that they are discussing, and (2) there is likely to be an underlying fear on Mrs Peterson's part of a loss of independence, and so presenting the issue of bathroom modifications as Mrs Peterson's decision helps to show respect for her as an independent adult.

Maxine also uses a positive politeness strategy here as well, however. In line 20, she expresses agreement with the importance of confidence (a word that Mrs Peterson has just used) and talks of confidence as a goal that she and Mrs Peterson share. This expression of common purpose, or even solidarity, is a positive politeness strategy, in that it is directed towards the listener's positive face. An important point to remember is that negative and positive politeness strategies are often used together, as shown in this particular interaction.

Reflective learning 4.5: Empathy, sympathy and facework

How do you gauge the effect of your displays of empathy on your clients or patients? What 'cues' or responses (verbal and non-verbal) do you receive, and do these influence your behaviour?

- Is displaying sympathy (as we have defined it here) an acceptable alternative to displaying empathy in healthcare consultations, or conversations between colleagues? How might a display of sympathy (rather than empathy) alter the dynamics of the interaction?
- Consider the words that you tend to use when making suggestions or recommendations to others. For instance, do you tend to adopt a blunt, direct approach, or a more tentative indirect approach? Do you adjust your strategies (ways of talking) according to whether the 'other person' is a senior colleague, junior colleague or patient/client? Give some examples of your lexical choices (choice of words) and discourse strategies.
- How would you explain your response to the previous question in terms of positive and negative face?

4.5   Summary

This chapter has focused on the ways in which people demonstrate understanding and respect for the feelings and perspectives of others. We have discussed the way that *empathy* is displayed in discourse, and how this varies according to the larger context in which an interaction is taking place. We have also introduced the linguistic concepts of *face* and *facework*, and have focused on ways in which people adjust their interactions to take account of the face wants of their interlocutors. In Chapter 5, we will continue to explore the notion of face, with a particular focus on ways in which interactions can go wrong when face needs are not given sufficient attention.

5   Polite, Persuasive or Pushy?

Concepts to be introduced, explored and applied

- Assertiveness and aggression
- Direct and indirect forms of communication
- Hedging and tentativeness

Objectives of this chapter
After completing the study of this chapter you will be able to:

- identify strategies in yourself and others which facilitate assertive behaviour and avoid aggression;
- understand when and why direct or indirect forms of communication are likely to be effective;
- analyse the impact of hedging and tentativeness on communication.

5.1   Introduction

In Chapter 3 we looked at various ways in which people respect the face wants of others when communicating with them. In this chapter, we will focus on interactions where there is an element of conflict, or where people have different ideas about what the outcome of the interaction should be. Where such conflict exists, one person may give way to allow the wishes of the other to prevail. Alternatively, they may stand up for (or assert) their own right to determine what they will or will not do. Depending on how this is done, it may or may not be perceived as a form of aggression by the other person. As we will see, the boundary between *assertion* (or *assertiveness*) and *aggression* is more complex than it first appears.

Although there may be some people who do not care whether or not they come across as being aggressive, many of us wish to avoid creating this particular impression, but at the same time we want to maintain a degree of control over our own actions and ensure that our best interests are not overridden by the agendas of others. We will explore ways in which people can engage in 'face-work' to strike a balance in these sorts of situations, and will focus on two particular strategies: *indirectness* and *tentativeness*.

5.1.1   Discourse as a focus for discussion

Interaction 5.1

Mrs Wilson has just seen a neurologist, Dr Lim, for the first time. After the consultation, she stops by the reception desk to make a follow-up appointment. Ms Conway is the receptionist.

1 Ms Conway:	Yes (.) can I help you?
2 Mrs Wilson:	Oh yes um (.) I've just seen Dr Lim and he's arranged
3	some tests and (.) he's asked me to come back to see
4	him again in four weeks
5 Ms Conway:	OK let's see [*looks at computer screen*] first available
6	appointment would be May the 7th at 2.15 (.) it's a
7	Thursday (.) would you like that one?
8 Mrs Wilson:	May 7th? But that's two months away (.) isn't there
9	anything sooner? Any day or time would be fine
10 Ms Conway:	That's the earliest I have (.) Dr Lim is booked solid
11	until then. Do you want to take it?
12 Mrs Wilson:	Well um (.) I'm <u>sure</u> he said four weeks –
13 Ms Conway:	– and as I've told you there's nothing until May, so (.)
14	what do you want to do?
15 Mrs Wilson:	well, could you check with Dr Lim first to see if that's
16	OK (.) he said four weeks but if he doesn't really need
17	me to come back 'til May then I'm happy to do that
18 Ms Conway:	[*looks displeased and picks up phone to Dr Lim*] Yes
19	I've got Mrs Wilson here (.) says she needs to see you in four
20	weeks but there's nothing available 'til May [*Dr Lim speaks*]
21	Friday the 5th? OK thank you [*hangs up phone*
22	*and turns to Mrs Wilson*] We can do Friday
23	April 5th at 8.45 (.) that OK for you?
24 Mrs Wilson:	Oh yes that's great (.) thanks so much for doing that,
25	I really appreciate it, and sorry to be a nuisance
26 Ms Conway:	[*types on computer and looks at monitor*] it's OK

Reflective learning 5.1: Passive, assertive or aggressive?

Mrs Wilson is clearly not content to accept the offer of an appointment in two months' time.

- How directly or indirectly does she communicate this to Ms Conway (in lines 8-9 and line 12)?
- How would you describe Mrs Wilson's utterance in lines 15-17? Specifically, would you characterise it as passive, assertive or aggressive? What reasons would you give for your choice?
- The two speakers here have competing agendas. What instances can you identify of positive politeness strategies (i.e. attempts to make the listener feel good) and negative politeness strategies (i.e. attempts to acknowledge and reduce the appearance of imposition) used by each speaker?
- Think back to your initial reaction to this encounter. Is Mrs Wilson 'polite', in your view? How about Ms Conway? How do your answers to the previous question above support your initial 'global' impressions of each speaker?

5.2   Submissive, assertive and aggressive communication behaviours

Calls for people to communicate in a more assertive manner at work (and other spheres of life) became common in the 1970s. This was accompanied by the rising popularity of 'assertion training' (or 'assertiveness training'), which aimed to help individuals (particularly members of groups traditionally more vulnerable to exploitation) to increase their interpersonal influence by expressing their rights in a forthright manner. Some perspectives on assertive communication have emphasised the importance of *self-expression* and *personal rights*. As Wilson and Gallois (1993) point out, however, communication takes place in real settings governed by *social rules*; focusing single-mindedly on self-expression without regard for the expectations and face wants of others is unlikely to lead to effective workplace communication. We argue that assertive communication is most likely to be effective when it is deployed as one of many tools in a person's communicative repertoire.

How can assertion be distinguished from aggression? According to Archer and Coyne (2005), definitions of aggression generally involve an intent or motive on the part of the instigator to cause harm to others. This intent to harm can be seen, for instance, in acts of physical aggression, as well as social or relational aggression (e.g. malicious gossiping). However, there are many examples of verbal behaviour that lay people would be likely to label as 'aggressive' but where a clear intention to harm is difficult to find. A more suitable definition for our purposes, therefore, may be one provided by MacDonald, which sees aggression as 'the hostile expression of preferences (by words or actions) in a manner coercing others to give in to those preferences (1978: 890).

The distinction between submissive, aggressive and assertive communicative acts is in fact inherently ambiguous, given that those who evaluate the encounters (participants, bystanders or third parties) do so from different points of view. Some may focus on what they believe was the *intent* of the speaker (or their own intent, if they were the speaker), while others may focus on the *verbal behaviour* itself. Others still may focus on the *social context* and tacit rules about who is normally allowed to say what to whom. For instance, a referee who warns a football player that he will be sent off the field if he commits a particular foul one more time would not normally be considered aggressive, while a player who warns a referee that he will seek to have him removed from the field if he makes another 'bad call' may well be seen to be behaving aggressively. The first example is likely to be described as a warning while the latter example may be construed as a threat, as warning the referee is not seen as part of the job of a football player.

Idealised views of communication in organisations sometimes assume that all participants have equal status and therefore equal entitlements to self-expression. Most organisations and institutions tend to have established hierarchies, however, which means that assertive behaviour from some members is likely to be accepted as part of the social order, while the same assertive behaviour from others is likely to be seen as challenging the social order. In some cases, individuals may wish to do exactly this – to challenge the entrenched systems (and sometimes people) which they see as perpetuating inequality, lack of respect and/or exploitation of certain members of the organisation. In other situations, however, individuals may be more concerned about maintaining their social relationships with others in the organisation, and may make interactional choices accordingly. There is therefore an ever-present tension between the desire to get along with others and the desire to have one's rights acknowledged and respected.

How might this play out in a healthcare setting? Consider the following interactions, which represent just three of an infinite number of possible ways in which this particular encounter could unfold:

Interaction 5.2

Lauren is the Director of Nursing (DON) at an aged care facility. Carol is one of four senior nurses who work at the facility, and is generally in charge of the nursing team during her shifts. Carol (privately) does not approve of Lauren's approach to the DON position, and sees her as aloof from the day-to-day concerns of the nursing staff. On this occasion, Lauren has asked Carol to come to her office to discuss some 'concerns' that she has.

1 Lauren:	Oh, hi um have a seat and I'll be with you in a moment
2 Carol:	OK thanks [sits down]
3 Lauren:	[types on computer for approximately 30 seconds, then looks
4	up at Carol] mm (.) sorry about that ah (.) what I wanted to
5	talk about was um (.) I had a look at the charts from
6	yesterday afternoon and I have to say I was rather um
7	concerned about the lack of detail that I saw
8 Carol:	Oh yes (.) um all I can say is that yesterday was an unusually
9	busy day with um Mr Hansen collapsing and Mrs Briggs
10	returning from hospital (.) I'm afraid we were all run off our
11	feet and (.) um even so most of the staff stayed back to
12	finish charting bu//t
13 Lauren:	//I'm aware that it was busy yesterday, but
14	unfortunately um the (.) auditors aren't likely to be sympathetic to
15	that sort of explanation, and you know they (.) they could look
16	back in the residents' files when they come next week and I'm
17	afraid we wouldn't look too good

(Continuation A)

18a Carol:	I understand, um, you're right (.) we need to um make sure
19a	the charts are properly completed (.) I'll have a word with (.)
20a	with everyone and stress this
21a Lauren:	mm hm (.) if you could make it very cle//ar
22a Carol	//very clear (.) and I'm
23a	sorry about this

(Continuation B)

18b Carol:	I agree it wouldn't look good, but um to be honest I think it'll
19b	happen again unless we have an additional nurse to do a half
20b	shift between 3 and 7 as we've (.) ah discussed with you
21b	before
22b Lauren:	I don't really want to get into a discussion about staffing
23b	levels now, it's more a question of accurate and complete=
24b	=I just
25b Carol:	thought that the auditors would be reassured if they
26b	could see evidence that we had identified a problem and

27b	taken concrete steps to address it (.) isn't that what they're
28b	looking for?
(Continuation C)	
18c Carol:	You mean you wouldn't look too good
19c Lauren:	I'm sorry? [appears taken aback]
20c Carol:	We've been telling you for months that we're short-staffed
21c	on the afternoon shift, but it seems you either don't believe
22c	us or don't care, so we'll be making it very clear to the
23c	auditors when they show up (.) at least they're likely to
24c	spend more than five minutes at the nurses' station

Reflective learning 5.2: Professional relationships

Consider Interaction 5.2 above.

- How would you characterise (in terms of the categories 'submissive', 'assertive' and 'aggressive') the verbal actions of each of the participants in the 'three possible endings' above?
- What factors would determine which of the three 'continuations' would constitute 'effective' communication in this instance?
- At what points can you identify potential threats to 'face' of each of the participants? What positive and negative politeness strategies are used to mitigate potential face threats?

5.3   Politeness: solidarity vs deference

In Chapter 4, we discussed the notion of negative and positive politeness strategies. Negative politeness (moves to reduce the sense of imposing on another person) is sometimes referred to as *deference politeness*. Politeness that emphasises the closeness between speaker and hearer and their common interests is known as *solidarity politeness* and makes use of positive politeness strategies.

In Interaction 5.1, Mrs Wilson persists with her request for an earlier appointment, and at various points uses negative politeness strategies to reduce the apparent level of imposition. Examples include:

- 'isn't there anything sooner?' (a question that acknowledges the difficulty of finding an available slot);
- 'any day or time would be fine' (indicating a willingness to be flexible);
- 'Could you check with Dr Lim first ...?' (phrased as a request, rather than an 'order');

- 'sorry to be a nuisance' (acknowledging and apologising for the imposition)

Mrs Wilson also uses positive politeness strategies, including:

- 'I'm <u>sure</u> he said four weeks' (indicating a desire to comply with Dr Lim's plan to Ms Conway, who is part of the team at this particular practice and might therefore be expected to appreciate compliant patients);
- 'Oh yes that's great (.) thanks so much for doing that, I really appreciate it' (expressing appreciation for Ms Conway's efforts and the outcome achieved).

In this situation, the hierarchical relationship between the two speakers is difficult to define, as one is an 'insider' and one an 'outsider' as far as the institution (a medical practice) is concerned. On one hand, Mrs Wilson is the client and some may feel that this places her above the receptionist in the practice. From another perspective, Ms Conway manages the appointment book and has ready access to Dr Lim, which gives her a level of control that Mrs Wilson does not have.

In Interaction 5.2, the hierarchical relationship between Carol and Lauren is much clearer, with Lauren occupying a more senior position in both the nursing hierarchy and the overall institutional hierarchy. Lauren expresses her 'concern' about the quality of the notes that nursing staff have made in the residents' files. From Carol's responses (in all three versions of this scenario) it is clear that Carol takes this as a criticism of her and her team, although a closer look at Lauren's actual words reveals that she has made her criticism (if that is what it is) in an indirect way. She does not refer directly to Carol ('you') or other members of staff or their actions, but comments instead on 'the charts' and 'lack of detail', and expresses 'concern' rather than (say) displeasure or annoyance. In linguistics, we would say that Lauren has not gone *on record* with her criticism. Nonetheless, Carol clearly understands it to be a criticism, and the subsequent turn (lines 13–17) seems to confirm that she is correct in her interpretation.

Why would Lauren express this criticism indirectly, rather than making it more direct? One reason may be that criticising another person is inherently face-threatening, and adopting an indirect approach tends to mitigate (or soften) the threat to the other person's face. Another reason may be that, by not going on record with her criticism, Lauren could more easily back away from it later if she had to, for instance if Carol appeared upset or angry. Lauren could then claim that she was merely making an observation and was not intending to apportion blame for the deficiencies that she saw. There is no guarantee, of course, that Carol would accept this *reframing* (see Chapter 3) of the remark as an accurate reflection of Lauren's original intention, but an indirect approach at least leaves open the option of reframing as a face-saving strategy.

5.4   Assertion and aggression through a linguistic lens

As we have discussed above, assertive approaches that focus narrowly on the rights of the speaker may not ultimately achieve the goals that the speaker has in mind. Speakers may therefore elect to adopt an assertive stance (i.e. standing up for something that they believe is right or important) but at the same time engage in facework to increase the chance of their message being heard and acted upon.

Continuation B of Interaction 5.2 is a good example of the use of face and framing strategies in the context of an assertive approach. Carol's response that the problem is likely to recur (lines 18b–19b) is potentially face-threatening, so she prefaces it with a statement expressing her agreement with Lauren (a positive politeness strategy). She then expresses her view that the solution will come from addressing staffing levels on the afternoon shift. Lauren appears to see this as a reframing of the encounter as a discussion/negotiation about staffing levels, and resists this reframing in her response (line 22b). Carol, however, persists in her attempt to pursue the 'staffing levels' frame (lines 24b–27b) by appropriating Lauren's concern about the healthcare quality auditors' upcoming visit, and *aligning* her response with what she takes to be the goals of both Lauren and the institution (i.e. satisfying the auditors). By emphasising the achievement of common goals, she is using a form of *solidarity politeness* in trying to persuade Lauren of the wisdom of her suggested solution.

The use of solidarity politeness in talking to a 'superior' may have very different effects, depending upon the institutional culture and the leadership style (see Chapter 11) of the person in the higher position. In some cases, it may be viewed favourably as a display of initiative and creative problem solving. In other cases, it may be seen as a failure to respect the institutional hierarchy by a person who evidently does not 'know their place'. In the latter case, the person in a higher position may be expecting a response that displays *deference politeness*, such as that which is exemplified in Continuation A of Interaction 5.2. Although Carol's response in Continuation A begins with a positive politeness strategy (agreeing: 'you're right'), its primary focus is on presenting a solution that does not impose on Lauren (i.e. she is not required to do anything), and it includes an apology for the 'imposition' that has already occurred. Continuation C is very different. Carol goes on record with a very direct expression of her feelings of frustration with Lauren and a clear statement of intention to 'go above' Lauren to have her concerns heard. Note that the pronouns 'we' and 'us' (lines 20c and 22c) do not include Lauren, and imply that Carol is expressing views that are shared by others. Note also the absence of any politeness strategies – either positive or negative – to mitigate the strongly face-threatening nature of what Carol has to say.

Reflective learning 5.3: Facework revisited

Consider the features of the broader context in which the interaction above might take place.

- What situational factors might prompt an individual in Carol's position to respond as she does in Continuations A, B and C?
- Have you been involved in (or witnessed) workplace situations in which one or more speakers have dispensed entirely with facework and expressed feelings of displeasure directly and without mitigation? What was the outcome in terms of (a) the issue under discussion and (b) the working relationship between the people involved?

5.5   Persuasion

In our everyday lives, we frequently advise or ask others to do, say or think things. In many cases, these requests or suggestions may be accepted by the other person without hesitation, but in some cases some effort is required to convince or *persuade* the other person of the merits of a particular course of action. Successful persuasion therefore requires that a *change in beliefs* take place, as no persuasion would be necessary if the other party was already convinced of the merits of what was being asked or advised.

Poggi (2005) conceives of persuasion as 'goal-hooking'. In order to convince someone of the merits of a suggestion or request, it is generally necessary to link what is being proposed to a goal that the other person has, or is assumed to have. Consider the following scenario:

Interaction 5.3

Brian and Roger are registrars who work in the same hospital and who are both preparing for their written fellowship exams. Brian is trying to persuade Roger to join a weekly study group that he attends.

1 Brian: why don't you come along tonight? I'm sure you'd find it
2   useful (.) we're going through past exam papers at the
3   moment
4 Roger: mm I'm not sure (.) I don't get home 'til almost 7.00 these
5   days and I really don't feel like going out again on weekdays
6 Brian: oh come on (.) you'd just be studying at home anyway, and
7   this is more fun (.) at least we can share the work a bit
8 Roger: well (.) I think I'm better on my own (.) I've never been into

9   study groups
10 Brian: just give it a try (.) you want to pass, we all want to pass, so
11   it's pretty focused you know (.) we don't just sit around and chat

Mark is one of the senior staff specialists on the unit where Roger currently works as a registrar, and is therefore one of his supervisors. Mark is also the leader of the study group that Brian has been attending.

1a Mark: you know about our Thursday night group, right?
2a Roger: mm yes (.) Brian was telling me about it
3a Mark: oh really? yes Brian's um been coming regularly (.) um I
4a   thought it might be something that would interest you (.) ah
5a   with the (.) um exams coming up=
6a Roger: =mm
7a Mark: have you ah (.) thought about coming along sometime
8a   perhaps?
9a Roger: Brian says it's excellent and- well, the thing is, I'm not really
10a   the study group type, I don't think um (.) and (.) um
11a Mark: oh it's totally up to you, no pressure, I ah just wanted to let
12a   you know you'd be very welcome

Reflective learning 5.4: The art of persuasion

Mark (the specialist) and Brian (the registrar) both think that it would be in Roger's best interest to come along to the study group.

- What differences are evident in the way that each of them tries to persuade Roger to come along to the meetings? Why might Mark and Brian adopt these different approaches? (There may be multiple reasons.)
- Do these vignettes demonstrate 'goal-hooking'? If so, what is the 'goal' that Roger is presumed to have, and how do Brian and Roger link this goal to the act of attending their study group?
- Can you identify specific instances in the vignettes above where facework is being done? What sorts of face-saving strategies are evident?

5.6   Convincing or coercive (persuasive or pushy)?

As Poggi (2005) points out, true persuasion involves changing the beliefs of another person. However, particularly where there is an unequal power relationship between the parties concerned, it is also possible to push people into doing something against their will, or at least where they are not truly convinced that it the best course of action. This is what is meant by *coercion*, and it is important to distinguish it from persuasion.

Because the potential for coercion is much greater when there is a difference in power or status (in an institutional hierarchy, for example), people in positions of power may be mindful of this and take care to mitigate any possible coercion. This is what Mark does in Interaction 5.3 above; he adopts a *tentative* approach in talking to Roger about coming to the study group. This is evident from a number of features in the discourse:

- A 'pre-invitation sequence': 'You know about our Thursday night group, right?' (line 1a). Although Mark has not yet invited Roger to come along, Roger is very likely to recognise that an invitation is coming. The pre-invitation gives Roger the option of 'preventing' the invitation if he wishes (by talking about his pre-existing commitments on Thursday evenings), or allowing him a little time to prepare a reason to decline the invitation politely when it does come.
- Devices to reduce the strength of the suggestion, e.g. 'I thought it might be something that would interest you ...' (line 4a). Words that preface the content of a message but seek to reduce the levels of certainty or force that accompany it are known as *hedges*. Common examples include 'I suppose ...' and 'I guess ...' and words such as 'kind of', 'sort of', 'somewhat' or 'rather'.
- An indirectly formulated invitation: 'Have you thought about coming along sometime perhaps?' rather than (for instance) 'Why don't you come along tomorrow?' This gives Roger the option to respond in terms of his consideration of attending a meeting of the group at some point in the future, rather than committing himself to attending a meeting on a specific day.
- The devices above are also ways of demonstrating negative politeness, i.e. of showing respect for Roger's right to make decisions for himself and not be 'imposed upon'. In addition, we can see other examples of negative politeness in line 11a ('it's totally up to you, no pressure ...'). Here, Mark goes 'on record' by stating explicitly that he does not wish to exercise any coercion. (This does not guarantee, of course, that Roger will not still feel a degree of pressure, as the suggestion is coming from his supervisor.)

Although much has been written on markers of tentativeness as a characteristic of women's speech (Lakoff 1973, 1975), both men and women use tentative speech frequently, and there is in fact a great deal of overlap between the genders in this respect (Leaper and Robnett 2011). While it is true that these softening devices may sometimes reflect a person's subordinate role where a display of authority might be seen (by themselves or others) as inappropriate, the same devices are also useful in simply 'being polite' and showing sensitivity to the face wants of others. In cases where they are used by those in higher positions in an institutional hierarchy, they can serve to mitigate the strength of suggestions or recommendations and serve as a tacit signal that the person concerned does not want to 'use' his or her status to achieve coercion.

We can also identify positive politeness strategies in Interaction 5.3. In the first part of the scenario, Brian's turns do not contain abundant hedging, tentativeness or indirectness, but they do emphasise solidarity and common goals (the hallmarks of positive politeness). In the encounter between Roger and Mark, Roger appears to indicate a wish to decline Mark's invitation politely (and indirectly) in lines 9a and 10a, and he prefaces this by reporting a positive appraisal of the study group that he has heard from Brian. This helps to mitigate possible threats to the face wants of both participants that might accompany the declining of an invitation, by making Mark 'feel good' about the quality of his study group, as appraised by one of the group's participants.

Reflective learning 5.5: Politeness

> Can you think of colleagues whose interactions are often characterised by tentative speech?
>
> - Would you characterise these individuals as unassertive or simply as polite communicators? What elements in their discourse and social behaviours help you to make this distinction?
> - Consider some of the individuals who occupy senior positions in your organisation? Do they tend to mitigate the influence of their status in the way that they speak, or do they tend to express themselves with few markers of tentativeness? What individual differences have you observed?

5.7   Summary

In this chapter, we have looked at the ways in which concepts such as assertiveness and aggression can be understood from a linguistic point of view. We have also explored the way in which communication in professional contexts involves the concurrent need to attend to 'face wants' through the performance of 'facework' throughout the interaction. This further highlights the fact that communication is much more than simply exchanging information, one of the central themes of this book. Chapter 6 will introduce a range of individual and contextual factors that can impact upon communication in healthcare settings, and will look in detail at the ways in which individuals seek to 'manage' the impression that others form of them, through their discoursal choices.

6 Projecting an Identity to Others

Concepts to be introduced, explored and applied

- Impression management
- Contextualisation cues
- Impact of cultural differences on interactions
- Recontextualisation
- Interdiscursivity

Objectives of this chapter
After completing the study of this chapter you will be able to:

- understand the concept of impression management as it relates to interlocutors;
- recognise 'contextualisation cues' used by speakers to channel their interlocutors' interpretations of what they say;
- identify the impact of cultural factors on the management and formation of impressions;
- appreciate the ways in which different ways of talking about and acting on the world influence each other through the processes of recontextualisation and interdiscursivity.

6.1 Introduction: impression management

The impressions that we form of individuals, and of particular occupational, ethnic or cultural groups, are (often) based on many factors. One of the important factors is the interactions that we have with people, and our perceptions of their characters as reflected in their discourse styles. In healthcare settings, such impressions may be formed in just a few minutes (for instance, where a patient and doctor 'on call' interact briefly but then have no further involvement with each other). At the other end of the spectrum, they may be the result of years of working together closely as colleagues, or in a therapeutic relationship. In either case (and in all between) we are continually forming and reshaping our impressions of those whom we encounter in our social and professional lives. At times, we may go into an encounter with preconceived notions of what the other person will 'be like', based on what we have heard or experienced about people from a particular occupational category or ethnic group.

The term 'impression management' was first used by Goffman in his pioneering work *The presentation of self in everyday life* (1959). According to Goffman, it describes 'the way in which the individual in ordinary work situations presents himself and his activity to others, the ways in which he guides and controls the impression they form of him, and the kinds of things he may and may not do while sustaining his performance before them' (p. xi). While Goffman approached the concept of self-presentation from a social psychological perspective, his work has also been picked up by those working within linguistic (specifically discourse) frameworks. The concept of impression management has been used, for instance, in the analysis of cross-cultural encounters in business meetings (Bilbow 1997) as well as the performance of candidates in job interview contexts (Lipovsky 2006) and spoken-language assessments (Luk 2010). Bilbow provides the following comprehensive explanation of the concept:

> Impression management is ... a bipartite process whereby speakers project, on the basis of their impression managing style, impressions of themselves through their discourse, and hearers interpret this discourse and create certain impressions of speakers, impressions that may or may not be at odds with the impressions speakers think they are projecting. (Bilbow 1997: 465)

When interacting with others, a person will always project a particular impression of him- or herself. While this may be done at a subconscious level in many cases, some individuals will show higher levels of self-awareness and concern for the impression that they project to others. In such cases, they will attempt to *manage* actively the impression that they are 'putting across'. This often involves moves that are intended to steer the interaction in particular directions and prevent the interaction from proceeding in other directions. Thus, as Luk (2010) points out, discourse management becomes a form of impression management. An interlocutor will generally be attending to the message that the speaker is conveying, but will also be simultaneously forming an impression of the speaker or, if the speaker and hearer are already known to each other, adjusting their impressions. Importantly, however, the impression that is being projected, consciously or not, by the speaker will be received through what

Bilbow (1997) refers to as the hearer's 'filter'. This filter will be influenced by previous experiences, as well as a range of factors that include age, gender, culture, ethnicity, language background, educational background, occupation and socio-economic status. All of these are elements of the World of Communication model, which we discussed in Chapter 1. Finally, individual differences at the level of personality and character will also have a profound influence on the way that such impressions are 'filtered'. These differences include patience, tolerance and sensitivity to the needs of others. The result is that the impression that is formed may or may not correspond to the intentions of the speaker.

Perhaps the most fascinating aspect of examining interactional discourse is that it is – by nature – interactive. As we have seen in Chapter 3, participants are often continually adjusting their footings (i.e. the alignments that they take up to the other participants) as the interaction unfolds. Some of these footing changes may serve to 'adjust' the impression that a speaker is projecting in the course of an encounter. Importantly, the responses of the other participant(s) often contain clues about the impressions that they are forming of the speaker, and speakers may then adopt moves which seek to adjust or correct the impressions that they believe are being formed.

Two caveats are needed at this point, however. The first is that the clues that come back to the speaker are again received through the speaker's own filter. This, together with the fact that the clues may be subtle or ambiguous (to begin with), can make them difficult to interpret – or even detect. The second point to bear in mind is that individuals vary in the degree to which they are sensitive to the impressions that they make on others, and indeed in the degree to which they are concerned about the impressions that they project.

6.1.1 Discourse as a focus for discussion

The following three interactions are extracts of data of two nurses assessing the health needs of patients (from S. Candlin 1997a).

Interaction 6.1

1	Nancie:	do you have hobbies or do you go to clubs, do you have
2		a circle of friends (...)
3	Mrs G:	no I have a circle of friends
4	Nancie:	yes and you see them fairly regularly
5	Mrs G:	yes almost daily someone calls on me
6	Nancie:	so you don't feel isolated
7	Mrs G:	no
8	Nancie:	do you smoke?
9	Mrs G:	no

10 Nancie:	do you drink alcohol
11 Mrs G:	in here (.) a lady that's in here and I have a tiny sherry each
12	evening before dinner but no I'm not a drinker, not to any
13	extent
14 Nancie:	I'll just put down one sherry a day
15 Mrs G:	but small, very small

Interaction 6.2

1 Mrs D:	I've gone down very quickly since I seemed to lose me sight,
2	me hearing a lot and I find that I can't concentrate like I
3	used to
4 Lydia:	yes it would be putting a limit on things that you could and
5	couldn't do, wouldn't it
6 Mrs D:	well I can't
7 Lydia:	so you can't have anything to occupy yourself with
8 Mrs D:	well I can't write to my friends very often and when I do I
9	wonder if they'd be able to read the letter when I get it
10	done
11 Lydia:	right, so
12 Mrs D:	but I'm grateful to be here
13 Lydia:	that's right
14 Mrs D:	and I cause as little trouble as possible I don't think I'm a
15	difficult patient
16 Lydia:	no I wouldn't say that you were neither, there's no worries
17	there (.) so you know you said you were always feeling tired
18	so does that slow you down a lot, so do you how's your sleep
19	been (.) because you've been so tired do you find you're
20	sleeping a lot more?
21 Mrs D:	oh well I take very strong sleeping tablets
22 Lydia:	and then do you sleep well?
23 Mrs D:	yes I usually do (...) but the heat has been absolutely
24	unbearable
25 Lydia:	it has been lately hasn't it been quite hot even at night
26 Mrs D:	the heat doesn't make any of us feel any better I'm afraid
27 Lydia:	no it doesn't
28 Mrs D:	still, you can always see somebody worse off than yourself

Interaction 6.3

1 Mrs Y:	I was made um (...) er (...) what do you call it of the [*name of*	
2	*organisation*]	
3 Sara:	oh president (...)	
4 Mrs Y:	no	
5 Sara:	or secretary	
6 Mrs Y:	oh yes and the group president	
7 Sara:	oh right so you were very involved yes	
8 Mrs Y:	yes I was (...)	
9 Sara:	so you were a good cook and could sew and (...)	
10 Mrs Y:	I used to take (..) I used to be the president at conferences	
11	I used to have hundreds of women there	
12 Sara:	right yeah yeah do y//ou	
13 Mrs Y:	//I've got the proof of it here	
14 Sara:	are you a good cook were you a good cook in those	
15	days?	
16 Mrs Y:	oh I think my sons are a better cook than I am	
17 Sara:	oh are they that's wonderful that you taught them	
18 Mrs Y:	I tell you what they used to do when they were boys,	
19	whatever I was doing they'd want to do you see	
20 Sara:	right right	
21 Mrs Y:	so they can sew they can knit they can (...) do everything	
22 Sara:	great you were ahead of your time weren't you, teaching your	
23	sons things like that, that's wonderful	
24 Mrs Y:	oh when we were on the farm I used to drive the harvester	
25	and a tractor (...) all those things	

6.2   Impression management

In Interaction 6.1, Mrs G responds to the nurse's questions regarding her social contacts and smoking, briefly and succinctly. When asked about her alcohol consumption, however, she prefaces her response with contextualising information, rather than simply answering 'yes' and waiting to be asked how much she drinks in a follow-up question. Her answer serves to create a *picture* of someone who drinks a small amount of alcohol in a social setting, even saying explicitly, 'I'm not a drinker' (line 12). Nancie responds by feeding back to Mrs G what she is writing down on the assessment form ('one sherry a day'), to which Mrs G replies 'but small, very small' (line 15). While it is possible that Mrs G simply wishes to ensure that the 'record' is as accurate as possible, it is also quite likely that she is concerned that without the contextualising information, 'one sherry a day' (line 14) may present an impression of her that is at odds with that which she wishes to project. Goffman (1959: 45) points out that where people present themselves to others, their performances tend to 'incorporate and exemplify the officially accredited values of society'. Mrs G belongs to a society that sanctions the consumption of alcohol in small amounts in social settings, and her 'presentation' of her alcohol consumption fits this pattern. As the interview takes place in a healthcare setting, Mrs G is likely aware that higher levels of alcohol consumption would be seen as a health risk, and may thus be concerned to present herself as someone who does not engage in behaviour that could damage her own health. Her self-presentation is therefore consistent with the moral values of the larger society, as well as the health values of the institution.

Interaction 6.2 also illustrates a performance that appears to accommodate (in Goffman's words) the 'officially accredited values of society'. The healthcare setting makes it possible (and indeed desirable) for patients to speak frankly and openly about illnesses, symptoms and other sources of discomfort or concern, and their emotional reaction to these. However, individuals who become consumed by health complaints to the degree that they seem unable to talk about anything else may be seen (sometimes unfairly) as complainers, a label with generally negative connotations in both healthcare settings and society at large. Interestingly, Mrs D punctuates her accounts of her current condition with statements that serve to mitigate her health complaints. By expressing (a) gratitude for the care that she receives (line 12), (b) a desire not to be difficult or cause unnecessary trouble (lines 14–15) and (c) an awareness that others may be 'worse off' (line 28), Mrs D is able to manage the impression that she projects. This image is, in part, that of someone who is sensitive to the needs and difficulties of others despite her own health problems. Interaction 6.3 illustrates the way in which a speaker receives signals from an interlocutor which provide clues about the impression that is being created. Subsequent turns can then be directed at correcting the impression so it is more aligned with that which the speaker wishes to create. When Mrs Y in Interaction 6.3 talks of being the group president of a particular women's organisation, the nurse interviewing her responds by asking her about her cooking and sewing skills (line 9). Interestingly, Mrs Y's next turn does not address the question of cooking or sewing skills at all, but recontextualises her leadership role in the organisation concerned ('I used to be the president at conferences ... I used to have hundreds of women there'). When Sara asks again whether she was a 'good cook' (line 14), Mrs Y comments that her sons are probably better cooks than she is, steering the conversation to one in which Mrs Y comes across as a woman who was 'ahead of her time' in challenging traditional gender roles. Although it is difficult to say with certainty, it appears that Mrs Y moves to 'correct' the image of herself as a woman who can cook and sew well, and when Sara's impression of her is reflected back as 'a woman ahead of her time', Mrs Y seems much happier to reinforce this image.

6.2.1   Contextualisation cues and inter-group differences

In each of the examples above, we can examine the impressions that the speakers project and can also look at the way in which this impression fits with what we have called 'accredited values of society'. In these examples, the nurses and patients shared a number of commonalities, in terms of their gender (female) and cultural/ethnic background (so-called Anglo-Australian). Despite the differences in age, there is still likely to be a shared understanding of societal attitudes towards issues such as alcohol consumption, gender roles at home, and complaining about one's health.

Owing to factors that may be both individually determined and group related, individuals will vary not only in terms of attitudes, values and perspectives, but also in their understanding and unconscious use of cues that signal the way in which utterances are to be interpreted. Gumperz coined the term *contextualisation cues* to describe 'constellations of surface features of message form that are the means by which speakers signal and listeners interpret what the activity is, how semantic content is to be understood and how each sentence relates to what precedes or follows …' (Gumperz 1982: 131). A wide variety of different linguistic forms can carry such contextualising functions, including changes in pitch, intonation or speaking volume, choice of words (lexis) or grammar (syntax), adopting a formal or informal register, using particular dialectal or colloquial features, formulaic expressions, and the sorts of opening, closing and sequencing strategies discussed in Chapters 2 and 3. Gumperz (1982) points out that the meaning of various contextualisation cues is only apparent (as the term suggests) in context.

6.2.2   Discourse as a focus for discussion

Interaction 6.4

Dr Jim Lawrence (Dr L) is the Medical Director of a hospital where Dr B is applying for a medical position.

1 Dr L:	Dr B? Thanks for coming in today, take a seat. I'm Jim Lawrence,
2	the medical director here [*extends hand*]
3 Dr B:	[*shakes hand*] nice to meet you, ah::
4 Dr L:	Jim (.) Jim Lawrence
5 Dr B:	ah Dr Jim, nice to meet you
6 Dr L:	Nice to meet you too. Did you have any trouble finding the
7	building?
8 Dr B:	This building? [*looks puzzled*] No (..) I just read the sign outside
9 Dr L:	ah (.) good. OK um thanks for your application for the RMO
10	position (.) I see you've just got your provisional registration to
11	work in Australia

12 Dr B:	Yes
13 Dr L:	but the last medical position you had was five years ago, just
14	before you immigrated
15 Dr B:	that's right
16 Dr L:	OK um so could you (.) perhaps you could tell me a little about
17	what you've been doing since coming here?
18 Dr B:	[*looks puzzled*] well I couldn't do anything (.) I mean without
19	registration it is illegal to work as a doctor in this country, so now
20	I have got provisional registration I really need this job, you see, as
21	I'm very worried about losing my skills
22 Dr L:	yes of course but [*looks through CV*] I'm sure I saw (..) oh yes here
23	(.) um you're working in medical records at Greymouth Hospital,
24	and you (.) ah did an AMC preparation course last year?
25 Dr B:	oh yes
26 Dr L:	um could you tell me a little about that?

Reflective learning 6.1: Impression management

Although Dr B has arrived on time for his interview, Dr Jim Lawrence asks him whether he had any difficulty finding the building.

- Why might Dr Lawrence have asked this question (i.e. what purpose does it serve)? Do you find it an odd or unusual question? Does Dr B appear to find it an odd question?
- How might Dr Lawrence's second question ('perhaps you could tell me a little about what you've been doing ...') relate to the topic of 'impression management'? Do Dr Lawrence and Dr B seem to share (as far as we can tell) a common understanding of the purpose of this question?
- From this brief opening sequence, what sorts of impressions might Dr B and Dr Lawrence be starting to form of each other?

As we have discussed in earlier chapters, encounters (even 'formal' ones such as job interviews) often begin with small talk about non-threatening topics before the more 'transactional' topics of interaction are approached. Such talk has been said to 'oil the wheels' of communication by allowing participants to feel comfortable with each other and build rapport (J. Coupland 2000). However, not all cultures achieve such rapport through identical means. A person from the same cultural background as Dr Lawrence may well recognise his enquiry about 'difficulty finding the building' as a standard conventional opening which could be seen as a form of polite acknowledgement of the unfamiliarity of the complex to someone who is visiting for the first time. It is in fact (to those who share a particular cultural background) one possible variant of an extended greeting sequence. However, someone from another culture may not recognise the question as such, and may therefore wonder why it is being asked. Dr B's puzzled response suggests that he and Jim do not share the same understanding of 'what is going on' at this point in the conversation (recall our discussion of framing in Chapter 4). In other words, the signalling value of this particular contextualisation cue is not shared between them. While one could argue that what they are discussing is of little consequence, it could equally be argued that it does not help to get the relationship between the speakers off to a good start. Dr B may well wonder why Dr Lawrence appears to question his competence to perform basic tasks, while Dr Lawrence may wonder why Dr B does not respond to his efforts to put him at ease with a polite, friendly opening.

Interviewees who share similar cultural expectations with Dr Lawrence of the way in which 'job interviews' tend to unfold are quite likely to recognise his open-ended invitation to 'tell me a little about what you've been doing' as an opportunity to control the way in which they package and present their recent activities – in other words, to manage the impression that they project. Dr B, however, appears to take this question as a follow-up to the immediately preceding topic: the last medical position that he held before immigrating to Australia. His response suggests that he feels the need to clarify that he has not been able to work in his profession since arriving in the new country, and the frustration and anxiety that this has caused are evident in his response. Once again, Dr B may wonder why Dr Lawrence appears slow to understand his situation, while Dr Lawrence may wonder why Dr B insists on focusing on his lack of medical work opportunities, rather than emphasising the efforts that he has made to achieve provisional registration and presenting these in a positive light. As we have discussed above, one function of contextualisation cues is to signal how an utterance relates to what has preceded it, and because the signalling value of Dr Lawrence's display question here is not perceived in the same way by Dr B, the question seems distinctly odd to him.

In the final lines of the interaction, it becomes clear that Dr Lawrence already has a copy of Dr B's CV, which outlines his recent work in medical records as well as the courses he has taken. Yet, as is common in job interviews, he still asks Dr B to talk him through these activities. It is often the case in job interviews that relatively little new 'factual' information is conveyed; those in the interviewer role may be more interested in *how* interviewees talk about their previous experiences, particularly in relation to the job for which they are being interviewed (see Gumperz 1992; Scheuer 2001; Lipovsky 2006).

We have discussed the ways in which contextualisation cues provide signals as to how particular utterances are to be interpreted, and the possible consequences that can follow when participants do not share the same understanding of the signalling value of these cues. One consequence is that participants may have difficulty managing the impression that they project because their contributions are not always understood as they intend them to be. In the interaction above, the impressions that Dr Lawrence and Dr B are forming of each other are unlikely to be the impressions that each of them would ideally wish to project. The inter-action above involved what is generally referred to as 'cross-cultural' or 'inter-cultural' communication, where participants have been socialised into cultures that are clearly different. As Tannen (1989) points out, however, we can see other intergroup differences as part of a broader notion of 'culture'; these might include differences in age, gender, social class, education, religion, and family norms.

Earlier in this chapter, we examined some instances in which speakers sought to 'recontextualise' information in an apparent attempt to correct impressions – or possible impressions – that were being formed about them. On another level, however, we are constantly recontextualising material when we communicate, as much communication involves taking elements from one communicative setting or event and presenting them in another. These elements can include what could be considered 'factual information' (for example, when reporting a radio weather forecast that one has heard to a friend). Linell points out that the elements transferred from one context to another may be much vaguer and broader, such as 'general attitudes, ways of thinking, ways of laying out or understanding patterns of discourse' (1998: 148). Scheuer (2001) notes that applicants bring to job interviews discourses from various spheres of the private and professional lives, and a successful interview performance can depend in part on the appli-cant's ability to recontextualise these discourses so that they align with the values and expectations of the interviewers.

In Interaction 6.4 above, Dr B's frustration at the time it has taken to gain registration in Australia is evident. From one perspective, his disclosure that he is worried about losing his skills and that he 'really needs' this job seems a frank and honest assessment of his situation, and would be unremarkable in the context of a conversation with a friend in a similar situation. It is possible that Dr B feels that sharing this information openly will allow Dr Lawrence to see his plight and perhaps offer him the job out of a desire to help him. Dr Lawrence, for his part, seems interested in hearing Dr B *talk about* his work experience in Australia, and the details of training that he has completed (despite the fact that the basic information is already provided in Dr B's CV). This suggests that Dr Lawrence is interested in the way in which Dr B might recontextualise these experiences to present himself in a positive light from an Australian employer's perspective. For instance, he could demonstrate his proactive approach to overcoming the registration barriers by seeking out and completing relevant training, and by taking a job that gives him the opportunity to learn through contact with the health system in his new country, albeit in a clerical rather than a clinical role. Once again, however, particular approaches to the presentation of oneself in a job interview may be valued differently from one cultural context to another.

6.3   Professional discourse and interdiscursivity

The term 'discourse' can be used in a number of ways. Throughout this book, we present transcripts of interactions which for which we use the heading 'Discourse as a focus for discussion'. In these instances, we are using the term to refer to samples of 'language in use, as a process which is socially situated' (C.N. Candlin 1997: viii). Our analysis of these interactive events focuses most closely on the context of the immediate situation. However, as Fairclough (1995) points out, discursive events can be analysed at a number of levels, including the context of the immediate situation, the context of the institution, or the context of the wider society or culture. As such, the term 'discourse' can also be used in a broader or more general sense to apply to the range of communicative activities and practices associated with a particular institution, society or cultural group. Although the term 'institution' here may refer to a physical institution, such as a company, hospital or school, it more commonly refers to social institutions, such as professions. This means that we sometimes talk, for instance, about 'the discourse of nursing' or 'the discourse of medicine', just as we could refer to the discourses of a range of non-health-related professions (e.g. the discourse of accounting and the discourse of management). In taking this perspective, we are following a definition of discourse provided by Candlin and Maley as 'a way of talking about and acting upon the world which both constructs and is constructed by a set of social practices' (1997: 202).

Put simply, the term *interdiscursivity* refers to the idea that discourses influence, and are influenced by, other discourses. Because discourse can be conceptualised at many different levels of context (situation, institution, society, culture, etc.), it follows that these processes of influence (i.e. interdiscursivity) can also be analysed at many levels. Naturally, the boundaries between the 'discourses' associated with different professions are not always clear-cut. For instance, a general practitioner might see a patient who is experiencing stressful events in his life, and may choose to adopt a counselling role in the consultation. While some biomedically oriented models of medical practice might see this as an example of the doctor appropriating the discourse of counselling or psychotherapy (i.e. adopting a way of interacting that comes from *outside* her profession), patient-centred models of medical practice would likely conceive of the counselling role as an integral part of the discourse of medicine. Taking a longitudinal or historical perspective, however, it may become clear that 'counselling discourse' was (at some point in history) strategically appropriated by practitioners of 'medical discourse' (in some cultural contexts) and thereby gradually became an integral part of the latter. This example illustrates how interdiscursivity is an agent (and indicator) of social change (Fairclough 1995; C.N. Candlin 1997; Bhatia 2010), creating hybrid discourses that did not previously exist as distinct entities, or resulting in the evolution of existing discourses.

6.3.1 Discourse as a focus for discussion

Interaction 6.5

Speech pathology is a profession in which clinicians traditionally carried out assessments of a language (or languages) that they spoke themselves. With the increasing linguistic diversity in many countries where speech pathology is an established profession, many speech pathologists now work with interpreters (professional or non-professional bilingual aides) in order to carry out assessments of people with communication disorders who speak languages that the speech pathologist does not. The following extract is taken from a de-briefing session between a speech pathologist (Sandra) and Italian–English interpreter (Isabella) following a language assessment of a bilingual speaker with aphasia.

1 Isabella:	In the English I'm not sure if it came across=
2 Sandra:	=the grammar
3 Isabella:	that's why I (.) I brought that up (.) that in Italian (.)
4	it may or may not be, but I thought it was important
5	that you know, because 'we <u>are</u> in Sicily' (.) 'we <u>have</u> in
6	Sicily' (.) he could've meant to say 'we have a volcano
7	in Sicily', but it sounded from the way the conversation
8	went that they <u>were</u> in Sicily (.) so I wasn't quite sure
9	but it wasn't up to me to decid//e
10 Sandra:	//no no
11 Isabella:	so I let you know, but on those (.) those words like
12	*pasta scuitta and pasciuta*
13 Sandra:	yeah yeah
14 Isabella:	that was happening quite a bit (.) I tried to make sure
15	that came through with you on- (.) at certain times (.)
16	other times I wasn't sure what he was trying to say...

The extract above provides an illustration of the concept of interdiscursivity. The discourse of speech pathology naturally involves talking about language difficulties experienced by the clients whom they have assessed, since communication difficulties are of central relevance to what speech pathologists do in their professional practice. By contrast, the discourse of interpreting does *not* normally include offering a commentary on a speaker's message, or referring to patterns of difficulty that a client is experiencing in attempting to communicate. In fact, in many professional interpreting contexts, such comments from an interpreter are specifically proscribed and would contravene interpreting codes of ethics (Roger and Code 2011).

In the extract above, however, we see the interpreter Isabella providing descriptive comments of this kind to Sandra (the speech pathologist). In doing so, Isabella is 'appropriating' some features of speech pathology discourse (e.g. talking about the speaker's patterns of language difficulty in Italian, and possible intended meanings of unclear utterances) in order to complement the interpreting that she has been carrying out during the assessment that has just been conducted.

Importantly, the interpreter, Isabella, in the extract above is not talking exactly like a speech pathologist would. She punctuates her commentary with indications that she is mindful of the distinctions between her role and that of the speech pathologist ('it wasn't up to me to decide', 'I tried to make sure that came through to you'), and with markers of uncertainty ('it may or may not be', 'I wasn't quite sure'). When relaying information more directly relevant to her own professional areas of expertise, markers of tentativeness are less evident ('that was happening quite a bit'). This debriefing session is thus an interdiscursive event, as the interpreter has found it necessary and useful to employ some features of discourse normally associated with another profession in order to help the speech pathologist to understand how the client's language disorder manifests itself in Italian.

It is interesting to note that this example of interdiscursivity reflects a wider social and institutional evolution; this is a hallmark of interdiscursive events, as noted above. In this particular case, the incorporation of features of speech pathology discourse into the contributions of the interpreter reflects the advent of a 'new' professional partnership in response to the need to provide access to speech pathology services for all members of an increasingly linguistically diverse society. This requires that participants reshape and realign their traditional discourses to respond to new challenges.

Reflective learning 6.2: Interdiscursivity in clinical practice

Consider a common 'event' that you participate in with other members of your profession. Examples might include a nursing 'handover' at the end of a shift, a medical case presentation, or a telephone discussion between two clinical psychologists where one is referring a patient to the other to continue care in another city.

- If one of the participants was an educated individual but not a member of your profession, how might this become obvious during the interaction?
- Would their 'non-member' status be evident only from a lack of specific professional knowledge, or might it also manifest itself in the way that they structure and organise their contributions (i.e. their discourse patterns)?

(cont.)

Reflective learning 6.2 (cont.)

- Give some examples of particular ways of talking or interacting that would be generally excluded (or proscribed) in your professional practice, but might be acceptable or even desirable in other professions.
- Can you think of examples of interdiscursivity in your own professional practice? How do these examples reflect (or even bring about) particular changes within your profession, the healthcare system, or society at large?

6.4   Summary

In this chapter, we have explored the ways in which speakers project an impression (intentionally or not) to others during the course of an interaction. We have also examined the ways in which participants might seek to manage the impression of themselves that they put across, by steering the interaction in directions that they feel will allow themselves to be perceived in a more favourable light. Contextualisation cues provide a way of 'signalling' to another person the way in which a particular utterance should be interpreted; however, such cues often rely on shared cultural assumptions, and their significance can therefore be missed (or misunderstood) in situations where people do not share the same underlying assumptions and expectations. Finally, we have considered the many levels at which discourse can be defined and analysed, and the ways in which different discourses (from various spheres of life) influence each other through the processes of recontextualisation and interdiscursivity. Understanding these phenomena provides one way of examining and understanding change and evolution in healthcare systems and professions.

In Chapter 7 we will consider how your discourse is determined, impacts on, and is impacted by the activities in which you engage as a health professional: the site of the engagement and the type of activities in which you participate.

7 High Stakes Interactions

Concepts to be introduced, explored and applied

- Sites of engagement
- Crucial sites
- Interviewing and being interviewed
- Critical moments
- Co-constructing interactions
- Metaphor in interactions

Objectives of this chapter
After completing the study of this chapter you will be able to:

- consider ways of eliciting information from another person;
- understand the concept of co-construction;
- recognise the alignments which a person takes in an interaction;
- appreciate the use of metaphor in interactions.

7.1 Introduction

It is a truism to say that we are all, on a daily basis, faced with new situations and with meeting new people. Within the healthcare workplace, where so much depends on first impressions, much is at stake in the first interactions between patients and professional carers. It is often in the first meeting that the seeds of a therapeutic relationship are sown, a meeting which can be demanding of the discourse of participants. How we present ourselves and how we approach the other person reflect the impact of our actions on the situation and our developing relationship, but is also open to scrutiny by others. This is especially the case in relation to the discourse we use to achieve our goals (see Chapter 1). Through our discourse, as well as through our actions, our professional expertise is always on 'the line' and open to the judgement of others. Similarly, what we say and how we say it demonstrates to patients, colleagues and others not only our professional expertise, but how we understand our relationships with others, our alignments with them, and indeed where we position ourselves – our 'place' within the institution – whether the institution of medicine, nursing, etc., or within workplaces/situations in those institutions.

But as carers, we are also always making judgements – professional judgements – as we attempt to build up a health picture or profile of our patients. What we come to determine at our various meetings can then be open to confirmation, or denial, in more formal assessment situations. Sometimes it is at that first meeting that we formally assess the person's health status and health needs – be it from the medical, nursing or allied health perspective. This activity of assessment, particularly for someone who has not previously experienced the need for healthcare within an institutional setting, is bound to be something of a novel experience and, as such, has the potential to add to the stress that the health situation itself may engender. Such an assessment, in which the patient is an active participant, is demanding of your social as well as your discourse skills if it is to identify accurately the patient's often complex health needs. Appropriate information must be elicited, realistic goals set, acceptable interventions planned, and desirable and realistic outcomes determined. Much is at stake in this early meeting, since not only is an accurate and rich assessment necessary, but the interlocutors must work towards establishing the basis of the therapeutic and trusting relationship on which all subsequent care depends (S. Candlin 1997a). Such a relationship forms a secure grounding for the ongoing relationship, so that on subsequent occasions, when interactions might take place in emotionally charged situations, the discourse becomes itself therapeutic and in no small measure is a key part of the caring process – for example when providing possibly unwelcome information. However, care includes not only physical and emotional care, and the manner in which to perform health assessments, but also plays a central role in delivering health education programmes, offering advice, counselling and advocacy (cf. S. Candlin 1997a). As healthcare workers, we operate within particular sites of engagement, that is, a site where numerous social actions/activities occur at a given moment in time. Scollon defines site of engagement as 'the convergence of social practices in a moment in real time which opens a window for a mediated action to occur' (2001: 147), and by mediated action he means any social action that is carried out. This social action could include not only discourse and technology, such as computerised technology (websites and the like), but also the use of semiotics: signs, signals, posters, flyers, etc. (see The World of Communication, Chapter 1). Now, in the total situation we can identify 'events' that we might call professionally crucial sites. Such crucial sites might include taking a health history, performing a health assessment or an investigation, engaging in a speech therapy, physiotherapy or occupational therapy session, Such sites often present particular critical moments (C.N. Candlin 1997). Critical moments refer to moments of significance in the discourse which have the potential to upset the status quo and as a consequence demand appropriate professional attention to restore the balance. These critical moments demand a high level of discourse skills, when, for example, we have to make strategic adjustments (such as a change of footing or engineering a subtle topic change) if we are to maintain a harmonious and cooperative therapeutic relationship. At such moments the interaction stakes are indeed high, whether we are performing a rich and accurate health assessment, giving new information which may include complicated instructions, delivering unwelcome news, or engaging in interactions which are brief and seemingly casual, but still therapeutic (Crawford and Brown 2011).

7.2 Discourse within the crucial site of health assessment

In the context of this chapter we focus our attention on a nursing health assessment as a *crucial site* which is dependent entirely on discourse. Information which is pertinent and appropriate must be elicited by the nurse in an interaction with the patient, not necessitating at this stage a physical examination or the use of equipment such as stethoscopes, etc. Assessments can, as in this instance, consist of addressing a number of domains: social, physical, emotional and spiritual, each consisting of individual 'items' to be explored; for example, within the physical domain the topics of diet, hearing, dental care, elimination patterns, etc. However what is important for us in this chapter (as in all other chapters in the book) is that you focus on analysing the discourse of the participants and how it contributes to the mutual achievement of goals, rather than to the macro situation of diagnoses and social (i.e. professional) actions in the form of therapies (see Chapter 2).

7.2.1 Discourse as a focus for discussion

Illustration 7.1

Sara (RN) talking to Mrs Y in her home in the community.

Sara: What we're going to do is just talk a little bit about you and you tell me a bit about what's happened to you since the nurses have been coming to you.

Illustration 7.2

Jane (RN) talking to Mrs C in her home in the community.

Jane: we're just going to be talking about you (...) and how you are how you manage at home
            that sort of thing. We've been coming to you for some few months now haven't we?

Illustration 7.3

Elaine (non-RN) talking to Mrs H in an aged care facility.

Elaine: so I'm just going to ask you the questions ...

Illustration 7.4

Naomi (non-RN) talking to Mrs B in an aged care facility.

Naomi: ... and I'm going to interview you if you don't mind (.) on a few questions about yourself.
            Is that alright?

Reflective learning 7.1: More on framing

Consider how the assessment situation has been introduced in the four illustrations above. Compare the discourse of each in relation to how the activity is framed, for instance:

- What does the framing tell you about:
  - the formality of the interaction,
  - power relations between nurse and patient,
  - minimising anxiety about the unknown?
- How do you think the choice of frame determines the conduct of the assessment process and the outcomes?

7.3   'Interviewing' and 'just talking'

We could say that the manner in which the assessment is to be conducted is indicated by the way it is framed (see the discussion in Chapter 3). Here we argue that the interlocutors' understanding of the frame sets the 'tone' of the activity and the rules of engagement. Ribeiro defines frame as 'Instructions which a speaker gives to the listener on how to understand the discourse message' (Ribeiro 1996: 182). Goffman (1974) (again see Chapter 3) views frames as the 'alignments' which people bring to each other in their interaction. Within the frame, speakers need to be aware both of the understanding and expectations of the interlocutor and also of the alignments that each takes in relation to the other within the interaction. Jones adds to this stating:

> [W]hen we speak we never speak the same language. We engage in a
> discourse system made up of rules and expectations and ways of seeing
> the world which we take for granted ... the notion of framing is grounded
> in the idea that people organise information and knowledge about new
> events, objects or situations on the basis of their experience (Jones
> 1996: 2).

Reflective learning 7.2: Introducing the encounter

Consider again the four illustrations above. Reflect on how different nurses in
different sites of engagement (with differing levels of education, experience
and expertise) have introduced and explained the procedure of assessment.

- How, for example, do Elaine and Naomi (who are assistants in
  nursing) introduce the interaction?
- When reflecting on Elaine's and Naomi's discourse strategies,
  think about how their introductions compare with those of RNs
  Sara and Jane.

In these discourses, we see that nurses frame the interaction in one of two
ways. Naomi chooses to 'interview you ... on a few questions[1]...'. Similarly,
Elaine chooses to 'ask you the questions', while Sara and Jane favour an informal 'talk', suggesting a casual everyday conversation. In an interview situation,
the interviewee has little control over the items, i.e. the topics, to be addressed.
The interviewer knows the questions, the interviewee is 'left in the dark', not
knowing what to expect. In an interview, Sarangi points out that 'we would expect to find an asymmetrical distribution of questions and answers, the interviewer initiating the questions and the interviewee providing the responses ...'
(Sarangi 1990: 127). Here we see the interviewer determining the topic
management – the choice of topic, topic change – and therefore has control of
turn-taking, determining the next speaker and the sequences of the interaction
(see Chapter 2). The nurse is in control and 'calls the shots'. This is in contrast to
the assessment which is framed as 'talk': 'just talk a little bit about you'
(Illustration 7.1) and 'just going to be talking about you' (Illustration 7.2), the
informality implying that they have equal control in the interaction. Furthermore,
the mitigating 'just' in each situation and 'little bit' in Illustration 7.1 suggests
that this is not a formidable procedure, but one which can be relaxed and

---

[1] Here we discuss 'interview' in terms used and understood by the users, and not as the tool
referred to in interview theory (cf. Talmy 2011).

informal. The overall theme is the patient: 'you', 'a little bit about you and you tell me about what's happened…', again mitigation is evident, this time in 'a little bit' (Sara, in Illustration 7.1 above); 'how you are and how you manage at home that sort of thing', using the mitigating 'that sort of thing' (Jane in Illustration 7.2 above). From the outset, both patients know what the conversation is going to be about, and as each patient is thematised, then they can assume they will each be familiar with the content, and can exercise a degree of control over what they need to disclose. They are active participants and as such *they* are building up the knowledge base of their interlocutor, in itself a means of empowerment.[2]

7.3.1   Discourse as a focus for discussion

Interaction 7.1

Sara RN is delivering nursing care to Mrs Y in her home in the community (data from S. Candlin 1997a).

827 Sara:	…so metamucil that's what you use for your bowels
828 Mrs Y:	yes yes that's right. Yes I put that on my porridge every
	…
831 Sara:	Right does that work?
832 Mrs Y.	Yes
833 Sara:	Does that keep you regular?
834 Mrs Y:	It usually does
835 Sara:	Right
836 Mrs Y:	But see when I had to take pain killing tablets for my (?)
837	the pain killing tablets make me constipated
838 Sara:	Constipated yeah. Do you drink lots of fluid?
839 Mrs Y:	Well I try to but there's not much fluid I like
840 Sara:	Oh isn't there because when you're on Metamucil you
841	need to have extra fluid with that
	…
844 Sara:	That's good right
845 Mrs Y:	And I always have a cup of hot drink first thing when I
846	get up in the morning
847 Sara:	That's good right. How much do you drink during the day?

---

[2] It is interesting to note that, after the interactions were completed, the information gleaned when the assessment was framed as an 'interview' was not as rich as that framed as a 'talk'. The interview frame resulted in posing questions which demanded answers that were not usually extended. Often the questions did not seem to relate meaningfully to the person's everyday life (S. Candlin 1997a).

848	Mrs Y:	Oh (...) I'm afraid I'm (...) I'm not a coffee
		...
850	Mrs Y:	it's the water we've got here. The water's terrible isn't it?
851	Sara:	yes it could be the water
852	Mrs Y:	yes yes I think it's the water ...
853	MrsY:	but I do drink (.) I'm not supposed to because I'm on a low
854		salt diet er (..) the packet soup you know ...
855	Sara:	right
856	Mrs Y:	I drink quite a bit of that
857	Sara:	How many?
858	Mrs Y:	Perhaps two or three ...
861	Sara:	And that's all you drink all day
862	Mrs Y:	oh no no no
863	Sara:	no
864	Mrs Y:	I try to drink coffee
865	Sara:	Right you don't like water obviously
868	Mrs Y:	Oh not this water but I love good water
869	Sara:	Have you tried boiling it and then letting it stand and
870		getting it cold?
		...
874	Sara:	Right because .
		...
877	Sara:	Right what about fruit juice?
878	Mrs Y:	Of course I've got dermatitis I haven't told you about
879		that
880	Sara:	Right yeah I've seen your dermatitis
881	Mrs Y:	yeah you know about that
882	Sara:	What about fruit juice. Do you drink much fruit juice?
883	Mrs Y:	er (..) I always have a fruit (...) ... because
885		of my bowels
886	Sara:	Right ... what about
887		about drinking some more fruit juice as a way of getting
888		your fluids up
889	Mrs Y:	Yes
890	Sara:	And that would help your bowels as well

After a further 14 exchanges Sara then returns to the topic of dermatitis previously introduced by Mrs Y.

906	Sara:	What's your dermatitis caused by

Interaction 7.2

Jane is delivering nursing care to Mrs C in her home in the community (data from S. Candlin 1997a).

54 Jane:	... and you have great support here from your families and
55	that don't you? One friend in particular and she helped you w//ith
56 Mrs C:	//you
57	know she took my washing=
58 Jane:	=still doing that? Are
59	you feeling a bit//stronger
60 Mrs C:	//I said to her I'm going downstairs and
61	she said you're mad she said give it (?) wait until Sister says you can come (?)
62 Jane:	yeah I think we're sort of winding down now you're becoming so
63	much stronger and your bowels are really good aren't they
64 Mrs C:	I haven't been today
65 Jane:	You had all that trouble with that diarrhoea which was
66	reason for you last couple of hospital admissions
67 Mrs C:	I never had a (?) that again
68 Jane:	No but apart from that you've been really well lately
69	most of your life
70 Mrs C:	yes yes I have
71 Jane:	This diabetes has that been it hasn't really been a
72	problem to you has it. That's been controlled by diet.
73 Mrs C:	I didn't realize until I was in hospital how serious it was
74	I thought it was (?)
75 Jane:	But all that diarrhoea made a difference
76 Mrs C:	And the (***) the (***) what do you call it (***) the (***)
77	sp (****) oh what's the other disease that goes with it
78	when you go up and down? Blood pressure
79 Jane:	Right that was affected was it?

From a discourse organisational viewpoint neither Mrs Y (Interaction 7.1) nor Mrs C (Interaction 7.2) is consciously involved in the task of assessment, and yet, as you will see in Interaction 7.2, the discourse of Mrs C demonstrates that she also introduces and reintroduces topics (e.g. line 76). Jane encourages disclosures so that the assessments are in-depth, rich and meaningful both to Mrs C and also to Jane (lines 71–72), who is able to plan appropriate care and interventions. This situation supports the view of Faulkner (1992), who proposes that, given the opportunity, the patient will volunteer information which is perceived to be significant, information which would not of necessity have been elicited in a strict question/answer sequence. The initial choice of frame can determine the discourse behaviours of participants for the whole interaction and the consequent quality of the assessment. Illustration 7.1 is an extract of the interaction between Sara and Mrs Y where Sara has framed the assessment as 'just talk'.

Reflective learning 7.3: Aspects of Conversation Analysis and framing in clinical practice situations

Consider the discourse in Interaction 7.1 not only as a means to enhance your learning in this chapter, but also as an opportunity to consolidate prior learning. Then refer back to concepts discussed in previous chapters.

- What types of sequences of turns can you identify as discussed in Chapter 2?

In Chapter 4 we discussed the notion of a person's 'face'.

- Reflect on how you believe that Sara's face is threatened during the interaction? What strategies does Sara adopt to save her own face and at the same time save and enhance Mrs Y's face?
- From your professional practice experiences, how have patients demonstrated their alignment (or not) with the institution? How were such situations handled - and with what effects?

Reflective learning 7.4: Crucial sites and critical moments

Reflect on the discourse in Interaction 7.1 and what you identify as the crucial site.

- Similarly can you identify a critical moment in the discourse?
- Think about how this critical moment is managed by the participants so that the focus of the activity is maintained, for example:
  - what strategic adjustments are made within the discourse;
  - at what point is the focus resumed and balance restored;
  - how is this received by the interlocutor?
- In what sense can Mrs Y and Sara be said to be aligning with the institution?

7.4   The use of metaphor

In Interaction 7.1, we see that the interaction is essentially *co-constructed* between nurse and patient. While Sara is aware of her own goals, she listens to Mrs Y's contributions, obviously regarding them as being meaningful to Mrs Y and in line with the goals of assessment. Sara guides the interaction to achieve the assessment goals, taking her cues from Mrs Y's contributions. Statements are made, questions asked, responses given, usually around the same topic, apart from a sudden change of topic by Mrs Y (line 878) from elimination patterns and fluid intake to dermatitis – a change which appears to have no obvious connection with the previous turns. We can say that this constitutes a *critical moment* which demands quick thinking by Sara, who must keep her eye on the goal so that the momentum of prior turns is maintained and understanding is achieved by Mrs Y. This understanding is essential if behaviour change in the form of increasing fluid intake is to occur (S. Candlin 2002). However, understanding cannot be taken for granted; it is something which must be 'worked at' by Sara who, in line 882, makes a suggestion which seems to be only partially understood by Mrs Y. For example, in line 883 Mrs Y picks up the importance of fruit but not juice. Her point of reference is 'my bowels'. Sara then repeats the topic of juice 'as a way of getting your fluid up' (lines 877–88). Only when Mrs Y agrees with Sara about her fluid intake does Sara refer back to the topic which is of obvious concern to Mrs Y (line 890). At this point, Sara returns to the topic of dermatitis, eliciting the advice given by Mrs Y's doctor and re-enforcing it. She not only achieves her professional goals, but also her discourse goals in that a *coherent interaction* is maintained (see Chapter 9); topic management strategies are successful as is the sequential organization of turns. What this achieves, then, overall is a harmonious and co-constructed interaction.

7.4.1   Metaphor

Note the manner in which, in the discourse of Sara and Mrs Y, *metaphors* are utilised. It seems that their use serves as a strategy by which the speaker (Sarah) accommodates her discourse to the interlocutor (Mrs Y). Whether these metaphors are adopted consciously as an accommodation strategy is a moot point, since many such metaphors are used in ordinary everyday speech and barely recognised as such by speakers. We need to explore metaphors further, turning first to the definition of metaphor provided by Burke and then to the work of Cameron (2010)

Burke (1945: 503) describes metaphor as: *a device for seeing something in terms of something else*. There are some problems with such a definition, however, as Cameron makes clear, principally because it fails to capture the richness of metaphor in action. She presents compelling evidence (Cameron 2010) for the need for a multidimensional view of metaphor: linguistic, embodied, cognitive, affective, socio-cultural, dynamic. We are particularly concerned here with metaphor as used by people engaged in specific social interactions – in effect 'discourse' in action.[3] Some might talk about political discourse, feminine discourse, nursing discourse, health discourse. But as our discussion develops, you will see that any such overarching category label masks the complexities of discourse practice in the caring context, since it risks not capturing the richness and the essence of the interaction of individual human beings in specific contexts. Much of this human action is created by the use of what Cameron refers to as *linguistic metaphor*, defining the term as something that is signalled by the arrival of 'something else', i.e. a word or phrase which contrasts with the discourse at that point (Cameron 2010: 4). We note, for example, incongruences where, for example, a pension fund is said to be in a 'healthy position', a person is reckoned to be 'all at sixes and sevens' or whose head is 'all fuzzy'. We seem rarely to reflect on this incongruence, so used are we to what can be regarded as ordinary everyday 'talk'.

Further, we might not think of some metaphors as being embodied where, as in much of our conversation, what we say in our discourse is accompanied by the non-verbal aspect of a communication event: gesture, movement, facial expressions. However, when we talk of metaphor as being embodied, we do not necessarily *see* the non-verbal action; rather, we hear the lexical choices which describe an aspect of an event. The linguistic metaphor is only a part of what is happening in a social interaction. 'She took a deep breath' is understood to be a metaphor signalling preparedness for a stressful event, and derives from the physical action taken to summon up strength to cope with a difficult situation (Cameron 2010). 'Weeping buckets' is another example of a metaphor used to describe a physical action. Sometimes, however, the action is used to replace or accompany the words, for example the three-year-old boy who was repeatedly warned by his mother to 'stop doing that, you'll break your neck'. He soon learned to cut her warning short with a gesture that simulated a broken neck: a hand drawn from one side of his neck to the other!

The fundamental tenet of *cognitive or conceptual metaphor* theory is that metaphor operates at the level of thinking and links two conceptual domains. We see that moral/ethical behaviour is linked with cleanliness, 'cleaning up ones act' or a 'spotless reputation' where amoral is 'dirty' as in 'dirty tricks' (underhand, unfair) or 'dirty jokes' (mildly pornographic).

The idea of *metaphor as affective* is exemplified in the discourse of a social worker supervisor who, when needing to discuss the deficient practice of a team member, would say to the person in question, 'we need to have a little chat'. Or the nurse who was heard to say, when helping with personal hygiene, 'oh dear

---

[3] This is not to say that metaphor is not utilised in the arts: in music, for example, or works of art. But for our purposes here, we will centre the discussion on discourse, particularly within the context of healthcare

we're in a little bit of a mess' (Lawler 1991). *Affective metaphor* seems to be a useful tool which minimises loss of face and allows the interaction to proceed in a less threatening manner, downplaying statements that might cause distress.

Metaphors having a *sociocultural basis* are those that emerge over long periods of time across speech communities, or are generated by groups of people who spend time together in the same place. Such sociocultural metaphors can be exemplified in the (seemingly uncaring) discourse of two nurses who talked about Mrs Smith having 'snuffed it'. In fact it is a metaphor which Mrs Smith (an ex-nurse) was heard to use herself. Its use following her death was not disrespectful, but was used by carers who had developed an affinity with her and were using Mrs Smith's own words to 'lighten' a sad event. Metaphors having a sociocultural basis are generally understood by members of the community but, by their very nature, risk being exclusive and obvious only to the in-group. In making use of these apparently innocuous metaphors, as health professionals, we must ask ourselves whether in doing so our discourse excludes others: the out-group – the patient or family. Metaphors, however, need to be mutually shared and understood. They are never static but evolve over time as interactions proceed. They are selected, adapted and built on with subsequent metaphors, as one speaker/writer responds to another, develops an argument, clarifies a position or constructs a description. We can see this process at work in the interaction between Jane, the registered nurse, and Mrs C in Interaction 7.2, where the phrases 'great support' and 'getting stronger' are used. These linguistic metaphors refer not to the support of a physical structure, but construct a description of Mrs C's improving health state.

Reflective learning 7.5: Metaphor in clinical practice

Consider the text in the discussion relating to Interviews (Section 7.3 'Interviewing' and 'just talking').

- What metaphors can you identify and in which domain do you think they belong best?

Consider now the discourse in Interaction 7.2.

- What metaphors can you identify in the discourse of Jane and Mrs C, and how do they relate to the dimensions identified by Cameron (2010)?
- Consider how the use of metaphor enriches the relationship and therefore the discourse of both Jane and Mrs C.

(cont.)

Reflective learning 7.5 (cont.)

Reflect on your work situation and think of occasions where metaphor has been a feature of your discourse situations; for example:

- How did they relate to the dimensions we have discussed, particularly the affective and socio-cultural domains?
- What were the specific reasons for how you used them?
- Did they evolve as the interaction proceeded, and did their use enrich or impede the interaction in any way; for instance, were they mutually understood?

Jane appears to believe that Mrs C is improving, using metaphors that are mutually understood: a 'bit stronger' (lines 59, 63), acknowledging families and their 'great support' (line 54), but ignoring the metaphor 'you're mad' (line 61). Instead, she responds to the friend's advice (line 62) with the metaphor 'we're sort of winding down', allowing her to indicate a further sign of improvement with another metaphor, this time related to the patient's elimination pattern 'bowels are really good' (line 63), which Mrs C immediately attempts to refute: 'I haven't been' (line 64). Would you agree that much of Jane's use of metaphor is within the affective domain (e.g. 'a bit stronger')? We could propose that Jane is being positive and, by so doing, encouraging Mrs C, a strategy which she maintains through much of the interaction. Perhaps you think that the example 'bowels are really good' would come within the sociocultural domain. There are, after all, very few instances when discussion of elimination patterns would enter into everyday conversation, but are frequently heard in the culture of healthcare. But perhaps you would argue that it comes within the affective domain, since again Jane is encouraging Mrs C and, by talking about the subject of 'bowels' (often a taboo word) in a matter of fact manner (befitting nursing 'talk'), Mrs C's face needs are met.

7.5   Summary

In this chapter we have shown that at a given *site of engagement*, a high level of communicative skills become necessary for health professionals if they are to determine their discourse and professional goals: identifying health needs through the elicitation of often sensitive information, and in turn imparting information that is understood, so that the end result is the patient's necessary behaviour change to improve health. Implicit in the discourse of the scenarios above is that health goals will be mutually identified and agreed. We can make this assumption since we have seen how the patient aligns with the nurse's agenda, and how they both align with the goals of the institution (since health assessment is a professional activity aimed at identifying goals, planning and implementing care which will improve health). From the outset, we saw the strategic use by registered nurses of discourse which indicated the framing of the event. We observed the management of topics and the sequencing of turns which demonstrated smooth turn-taking with few instances of overlapping speech. As with a dance or a stage production, we saw each participant move in response to the other, and where this did not occur, the crucial moment was identified and managed with skill by the nurse so that the patient's face was maintained. The discourse was in effect co-constructed between interlocutors. Facework was demonstrated too in the strategic use of metaphor, particularly utilising the affective and sociocultural domains. We could argue that the developing relationships, indicated by the apparent willingness to disclose information, demonstrates a relationship of trust – an essential prerequisite if the patient is to be considered as a partner in healthcare.

Building on these themes and concepts in this chapter, we are now in a position in Chapter 8 to change our focus to consider how interpersonal relationships between members, not only of the healthcare team and patients, but also members of other professions, can be explored and described, in particular addressing concepts and themes in challenging situations, such as breaking bad news, and how interlocutors take up alignments and affiliate with the other person, recognising that these too are situations which demand the disclosure of personal information, and as such the stakes are indeed high.

8 Challenging Situations, Challenging Discourses

Concepts to be introduced, explored and applied

- Communicating bad news
- Risk-taking
- Alignment and affiliation

Objectives of this chapter

After completing the study of this chapter you will be able to:

- discuss the nature of bad news in various contexts;
- explore the nature of discourse strategies used to meet the demands of new events;
- identify strategies for delivering bad news: forecasting, stalling, being blunt;
- identify some sequences of conversation in news events: e.g. the news delivery sequence (NDS), perspective display series (PDS);
- understand the nature of tensions involved in aligning with a position, institution, person or group.

8.1   Introduction

In this chapter we will be introducing, exploring and applying concepts related to the 'breaking of bad news', with a view to determining the discourse processes by which this is achieved (cf. Maynard 1998, 1996). While we recognise that news situations occur in all manner of contexts, we are, of course, particularly interested in those which take place in the healthcare workplace because dis-course situations involving the delivery of news is not an uncommon feature of healthcare discourse. News delivery or, as we shall sometimes refer to it, the 'news event', as with most other utterances, does not occur in isolation but is an integral part of daily life, shaping and shaped by the individuals concerned. We argue that, in general, there are features which impact on the event, or are impacted by it, in that the event:

- occurs within a context, both localised within the discourse, and within the wider sociocultural-political context, and
- has a history, with news occurring as a result of some happening and is therefore part of a process.

The interlocutors are participants in the event as bearers or recipients of news, and, as with the news itself, their participation in the interaction is a significant part of their *lifeworld* since:

- each person is related to others within the local context and is impacted by the relationship – either as a deliverer or recipient of news, or as a co-participant, for example as a colleague;
- the event has outcome/s and, as such, is part of an ongoing situation;
- each participant brings their own perspective of the news which may have a bearing on their interpretation of it and therefore, potentially, on outcomes.

What we have found so far in this book is that conversations are highly structured and rule governed (see Chapter 2), with utterances occurring in regulated sequences, for example as with adjacency pairs or two-part sequences: a greeting being followed by an acknowledgement; a question by an answer and sometimes an extension of the response (making it then a three-part utterance). We have also found that discourse is usually a cooperative venture, so that participants are able to develop a shared understanding of the situation. The delivery of bad news, however, can be challenging for the participants since, by its nature, it can cause confusion for the individual. The discourse surrounding such events is complex and so, in an attempt to 'unwrap' this complexity, we will examine situations concerning the delivery of bad news and determine whether regulated sequences are present in its delivery and reception. This entails com-paring news events and how the breaking of 'bad' news is similar to, but also different from, delivering 'good' news. And here we are not making any judge-ment about what is 'good' or 'bad', but merely assuming that the delivery or receiving of information (or news) can be considered positively or negatively by the deliverer or recipient.

Maynard makes the point that 'news of a particular kind, is a conditional matter, dependent on the actions and responses of participants in conversational interaction' (Maynard 1997: 94). Because news delivery events take place within the context of the daily life of individuals, we need to acknowledge that such news impacts in some way or another on the *order of the social world*. While it is to be expected that as a result of the nature of the 'news' tensions might arise within the situation, there are indications that the discourse partnership is nonetheless frequently a cooperative venture, with the discourse being *co-constructed* as each partner makes strategic adjustments in their discourse in an attempt to maintain the social order.

To cast light on some of the complexities of the discourse process involved, we will base our discussion on aspects of the theory of CA to help raise an awareness and understanding of our own delivery of, and responses to, news situations. We will identify the processes involved in delivering news items, for example the manner in which news is announced, the *preamble, lead-in* and *preparatory statements* which in turn lead to the news announcement. Importantly, we will identify in extracts of conversation where the *perspective* taken by participants is a factor in the news delivery and consider the impact this might have on the actual delivery of news. We will consider too the style of news delivery and whether the deliverer engages in *stalling* the information/disclosure, is *blunt* and direct, or *forecasts* the news gently. We will then address news delivery sequences (NDS) as discussed by Maynard (1997) before the *realisation* of the news by the recipient occurs. What we will argue is that often there is an *order* which can be identified in news delivery. We have emphasised throughout the text, and particularly in Chapter 1, that the verbal content of the message is not the totality of the message; this is of particular importance when we are delivering bad news. We need to consider the effects of non-verbal aspects of communication and to the use of space, whether consciously or unconsciously employed, in the breaking of news. How does the delivery of the message, both verbal and non-verbal, impact on the facilitation of the realization of the news, or indeed on the relationship between the deliverer, recipient, the news item and daily life?

A further point is that you need to acknowledge and understand the strategic use of the discourse of others, and the resulting responses of interlocutors, so that consciousness of your own discourse strategies is raised – a necessity if news is to be imparted with sensitivity, and you are to be prepared for both expected and unexpected responses in the process. As with previous chapters, much of your understanding will develop as a result of your own individual reflections as you work through the activities and analyse extracts of data from situations which focus on the breaking of bad news.

Reflective learning 8.1: Understanding the notion of 'bad news'

Reflect on a situation where you received what you consider to be bad news (not necessarily health related). For instance:

- Consider the total situation, e.g. circumstances that may have led up to the event, the place and time where you received the news, the people involved etc.
- Reflect on the immediate impact of the news, e.g.
  - what emotions did the news engender?
  - how did it impact on your life? How, in fact, was the order of your social world disrupted?
- How might the news have been given differently to effect different outcomes?
- Now think about the individual differences between you and the deliverer of the news (for example, different sociocultural backgrounds, age, gender). How did these differences affect both the delivery and reception of the news?

(Here you might wish to refer back to the World of Communication model in Chapter 1.)

8.2   Issues arising in the delivery of news

The delivery of news can impact on the individual's life in a significant way, so much so that Maynard (1996, 1998) argues that the reception of *bad news* represents a *rupture in the fabric of everyday life.*[1] We can regard this rupture, or *disruption*, as a function of a (news) event which is 'atypical, unlikely, unpredictable'. As such, it can cause confusion and uncertainty. The recipient of bad news then has to orient to a changed reality, the response to which is dependent on many factors, not least being the perception by the interlocutors (or participants) of the *valency* or significance of the news. Is the news event always considered to be bad (or good) by both participants? And what stance does each interlocutor adopt to the event? Not only does the giving and receiving of bad news have the potential to cause emotional distress and confusion, but waiting for news can also cause anxiety and stress, as we can see in the situation outlined in Interaction 8.1 (see, for example Sonia's response in line 5).

---

[1] Similarly, of course, *good news* might also be seen as something that is out of the quotidian order, so that the predictable world of the person's ordinary everyday life is disturbed in some way, albeit positively, where the emotional response to the news can be happiness or even elation.

With so much at stake, it is important that we consider in our reflections the stance that each interlocutor takes to the situation and to each other, and how this might impact on the reception of the news. Maynard (1998) suggests that the deliverers of news have a responsibility for what they report. However, the response of the recipient, like the news itself, is not always predictable, since both interlocutors are influenced by individual differences, whether they be, for example, in the emotional, physical, spiritual, sociopolitical or cultural domains. We would argue that the attitudes of daily life and the socially organised practices of such life are a function of the values, beliefs and behaviours of the culture of each person in which attitudes and practices are developed and established.

Here it is important to recognise that we are taking a broader definition of culture – one that moves away from ethnicity as the one defining feature of culture – and, with Thompson (1990: 123), define culture as the 'array of beliefs, customs, ideas, and values, as well as the material artifacts, objects and instruments, which are acquired by individuals as members of the group or society'.

8.3   Some discourse strategies used when delivering news

8.3.1   Introductions to and pre-announcements of news events

When news is delivered there is usually some inclination/forewarning that something new is about to be shared, as for example: 'Have you heard the latest …?'; 'Oh have *I* got something to tell *you*?' While these statements prepare the interlocutor for a news event, they do not indicate the nature of the news. On other occasions, the news is foreshadowed such that the interlocutor is prepared for 'bad' news, e.g. 'Jane it's not good news I'm afraid …', or 'I don't know how to tell you this but …' Conversely, the deliverer might be heralding good news, e.g. 'Hey guys, have you heard about Jane and Pete – it's so exciting'. None of these pre-announcements invites the interlocutor's immediate involvement except as a passive listener. There is no suggestion that the news delivery itself will implicate the interlocutor as an active participant in the interaction, and there is no hint of the perspective that the giver of news will consider.

8.3.2   The perspective display series

From the outset, the holder of information may take on occasion a different approach from the above to the news delivery and makes strategic use of what Maynard identifies as the perspective display series (PDS), which he characterises as a 'device … (which) operates in an interactionally organized manner to co-implicate the recipient's perspective in the presentation of diagnoses' (Maynard 1992: 333). To take an example, the clinician, aiming to bring the recipient's perspective in line with his, will first need to know what the patient understands of the situation so that misunderstandings can be corrected and news can be 'pitched' appropriately. There is an immediate sense of the recipient's involvement in the interaction, and a sharing of knowledge and ideas. The patient is encouraged to offer his or her *perspective* on the situation – not only the understanding of the actual diagnosis, but of the wider view, such as the impact of the diagnosis on treatment. Often, this leads to the recipient of news volunteering information related to the impact of the diagnosis on daily life, and possibly the short- and long-term implications of the diagnosis and/or treatment. The strategies for *co-implicating* the patient will include confirming the recipient's understanding, which in turn might necessitate reformulating utterances, elaborating statements and offering explanations. Such strategies enable the doctor not only to understand the patient's perspective, but to tailor the information accordingly, so that the doctor's perspective is taken, thus effectively ensuring that both participants co-construct the conversation from a common perspective – the event being interactionally organised. The following interaction involving a physician, Dr David James, and the patient, Sonia, takes place in the physician's consulting room.

8.3.3   Discourse as a focus for discussion

Interaction 8.1

Sonia is a registered nurse with four children under nine, including a five-month-old baby and a toddler. She presents with a history of facial parasthesia extending across her shoulder and right arm, with a feeling of swelling and tightness around her wrist, a disturbed sense of feeling in her hand and fingers and a very poor grip. Her GP suggested that she might have 'a trapped nerve' but should see a consultant physician for his opinion, and she was duly referred to Dr James. After taking Sonia's medical history and performing an initial physical and neurological examination, the interaction continues.

1 Dr James:	Hmm Sonia now what do <u>you</u> think is going on?
2 Sonia:	Oh I've no idea except that my GP thought it might be a trapped
3	nerve. All <u>I</u> know is that with a family and a 6 month old baby, keeping
4	things together's almost impossible. I'm <u>terrified</u> I'm going to drop the
5	baby or something will happen and I can't <u>manage</u>
6 Dr J:	Yes that <u>is</u> a worry for you (....) you must have <u>some</u> ide//a
7 Sonia:	//no I
8	honestly <u>don't</u> I only know that <u>not</u> knowing is <u>horrible</u> //and scary
9 Dr J:	//well you <u>don't</u> have MS
10 Sonia:	I never thought I//did
11 Dr J:	//oh I thought <u>all</u> nurses would jump //to <u>that</u> conclusion
12 Sonia:	//no so what <u>is</u> it don't

13		tell me it's spondylitis
14	Dr J:	Now why would that worry you
15	Sonia:	Oh I don't know except that I have a dread of being a little old lady crippled
16		with arthritis like some of the patients I've nursed
17	Dr J:	You haven't got arthritis but (...) hmm what we'll do is look at the clinical
18		picture and do some investigations (..) send off some blood take some
19		XRays and do a lumbar puncture see if the CSF will tell us anything. Now
20		you said you were going on a short holiday this weekend so can you come
21		in overnight so we can do the lumbar puncture?

A number of significant issues arise in this brief extract; for example, you can immediately see that consideration is given to the wider context of the patient's life. Dr James is taking the patient's *perspective* (line 1) implicitly considering her social/professional world, and allowing Sonia to present what is important to her, the impact of her illness on her social and lifeworld, i.e. the threat ('I'm terrified', line 4) which her illness presents to the *social order* ('keeping things together', line 3 'can't manage', line 5). The conversation is cooperative, in that turns are offered and taken, with overlapping speech, when it occurs, being appropriate in that the responding overlap can be considered to be an attempt at reassurance (line 9) or a possible explanation by Dr James for his prior utterance – which might be interpreted as being gratuitous. By implicating the *perspective* of 'all nurses' (line 11), he is possibly attempting, in his explanation, to remove any perceived (and unstated) misunderstanding (i.e. of the reason why Sonia might conclude she has MS).

When we look at this approach to the delivery of news, we see that it is very much dependent on the *perspectives* which each participant brings to the situation. Dr James is aware of Sonia's professional background and is seeking to collaborate with her by attempting to implicate her *professional perspective* (line 1, and again in lines 6 and 11). What we have effectively done in this discussion of the situation is to frame the analysis of this extract in terms of the *perspective display series* (PDS) as we indicated above – as a device which 'operates in an interactionally organised manner to co-implicate the recipient's perspective in the presentation of a diagnosis' (Maynard 1992: 333). Sonia, however, is taking the *maternal perspective*, since her concern is, ostensibly, as much to do with the impact of her illness on her mothering responsibilities as it is on making a diagnosis (lines 3–5). Dr James responds with another PDS (lines 9 and 11) by returning to the *patient's (professional) perspective*, having first acknowledged Sonia's concerns. Following an apparent attempt to reassure her (line 17), Dr James then takes the *clinical perspective* (lines 17–19) discussing the need for investigations without committing to a provisional diagnosis.

From the patient's viewpoint, there is an obvious threat to the social order. She wants a return to her predictable world as is reflected in her wanting a diagnosis stating, 'not knowing is horrible and scary' (line 8). Dr James, knowing that he is not going to make a diagnosis at this point in time, manages the interaction by attempting to reassure her (lines 9 and 17). Recognising that her anxiety is probably unappeased, he immediately follows his attempt in line 17 with a strategy (dependent on Dr James taking a *clinical perspective*) which represents a step towards achieving a diagnosis.

Reflective learning 8.2: The management of news situations

After reflecting on Interaction 8.1 you might consider that there is no indication of actual bad news, in that there is no specific diagnosis. But in view of the patient's acknowledged fear, perhaps this is the (unstated) bad news. Maybe the thought of 'investigations' present bad news, specifically the need for a lumbar puncture, since a nurse would have an idea of what it entailed. Perhaps the need to spend time in hospital away from her mothering duties is indeed bad news for her.

- Reflect on these suggestions. What are your thoughts?
- Do you think that the doctor was making assumptions as a result of the perspectives taken?
- Consider how the interaction might have been conducted differently (particularly if different perspectives had been taken).

Now, from your professional and life experience, reflect on a situation where bad news has been given to somebody with different values and beliefs from those of the mainstream community.

- Following our analysis of Interaction 8.1, and particularly of the perspectives taken to co-implicate the patient, what comparisons can you make between the management of the situation you observed/participated in and that in the scenario? Specifically, did you observe a perspective display series? What were the effects of any PDS on the interaction? How was the interlocutor co-implicated in the interaction?
- How have you been prepared to deal with situations where you have had to deliver bad news to a person? What communicative actions did you take and what 'strategies' did you adopt?
- As a result of your experiences and your reflections here, how would you now approach such a situation?

8.3.4   The news delivery sequence

Clearly, the delivery of bad news is a communicative activity which demands skill and sensitivity if any negative impact on the recipient is to be minimised. This does not imply, however, that the news, in the short term, will necessarily be less painful; what it might suggest is that at very least taking a sensitive approach would not add to the pain of the news. What we can say is that the skill of sensitive news deliverers can be seen in the strategies that they adopt and the consideration they give to the variables we have discussed earlier surrounding the news event: the type of news, the culture, values and beliefs of the recipient, the awareness of the recipient of the situation, perception of the impact on the social order and so on. What is especially significant here is the manner in which the recipient is *prepared for* the news.

You can see from Interaction 8.2 how (as with the PDS) the participants construct the sequence interactively, where the discourse actions and responses of the participants indicate, firstly, that they share information about their world (see the first two exchanges), secondly, how the gradual unfolding of the news signals the valence of the news even before the news is actually stated. Both participants see redundancy to be bad news, but you cannot automatically assume this. Some people, for example, might welcome the news that their current employment has been terminated, and see the situation as an opportunity to begin a new life, or to explore other employment options, outcomes which neither the supervisor nor the worker share. Thirdly, we see a convergence of understanding as they recognise the particular effects that the information has for each of them (lines 19–21). Maynard (1997: 4) states that 'good or bad news as it emerges in the particularities of the conduct of those co-present to one another, like every other feature of a setting, is a "contingent accomplishment of socially organised common practices"' (Garfinkel 1967: 33).

8.3.5   Discourse as focus for discussion

Interaction 8.2

Giovanni works as a section manager in a manufacturing business and meets regularly with his supervisor to discuss work-related matters. He has been called in by his supervisor and assumes it is to discuss the work practices of his team.

1 Supervisor:	Giovanni come in (1.0) sit down. Look I must ta:lk to you about the
2	situation here. I've no complaints about your work far from it but the
3	truth is (0.2) as you know (.01) we've er not been getting the orders
4	in to maintain full employment

```
5 Giovanni:      I realise this (0.2) and I know you've been against laying people off so
6                does it mean we're going to change the way we do things?
7 Supervisor:    (1.0) It's er much more radical than that I'm afraid
8 Giovanni:      Oh? What are you trying to sa::y?
9 Supervisor:    I don't think you're going to like hearing this (.06) I certainly don't
10               like having to say//it
11 Giovanni:                      //oh no (.01) I can't believe what's coming
12 Supervisor:   (.02) 'fraid so. There's enough work for a few more weeks but after
13               that (.02) well we're up the creek without a paddle. I'm afraid I'm
14               going to have to release you next month but you'll get another month's
15               work on half-pay and of course I'll give you a good //reference
16 Giovanni:                                                //I can't believe this
17               two kids' school fees, a mortgage, sick parents and my wife only working
18               part-time (.02) never rains but // it pours
19 Supervisor:                             // know what you mean (.05) don't much
20               know what I'm going to do myself either when my turn comes and come
21                it certainly will
```

As we analyse the discourse more closely, we can see that there is a *pre-announcement* (lines 1–4) to the news delivery. Interestingly the supervisor appears to 'soften the news' by referring, in mitigation, to Giovanni's work practices. The praise can also be seen then as an indication to Giovanni that what is coming is no reflection on Giovanni's work ethic. The interaction work (lines 5–6) appears to be given more immediate salience than the actual news item, since it allows Giovanni to demonstrate his understanding of the situation and make a *news enquiry* (line 6) to which the supervisor takes another step in the *gradual unfolding* of the *news announcement*. The statement in line 7 we can consider to be another step in the unfolding, but this time indicating that 'bad news' is about to be broken – 'more radical than that'. It is with this response that we see the continuation of the *news delivery sequence* (NDS) This is a four-part sequence consisting of the *announcement, announcement response, elaboration* and *assessment*. The pre-announcement (lines 1–4) heralds the announcement which, interestingly, is not stated directly (line 9) but is immediately understood by Giovanni (line 11) in an announcement response. This then occasions the elaboration of the news by the supervisor in lines 12–15. The assessment of the situation is made by Giovanni (lines 16–18). In this extract we might want to consider the assessment as being a two-part sequence as the supervisor, after listening to Giovanni's assessment, demonstrates his empathy for Giovanni by affiliating with him (lines 19–21).

Reflective learning 8.3: Discourse strategies used in the breaking of bad news

From your understanding of CA, which we discussed in Chapter 2, consider the argument so far in this chapter and the manner in which we have displayed the turn-taking sequences. Now examine the lexical items and phrases in Interaction 8.2.

- How do you consider that these are used to herald:
  - a new turn;
  - the valence of the news being delivered;
  - an empathic display by the supervisor and his affiliation with Giovanni?
- How does the supervisor demonstrate his alignment with the institution?
- What indications are there, if any, of tensions experienced by the supervisor in his affiliation with Giovanni and his alignment with the institution (i.e. in that we can consider the supervisor to be the spokesperson for the institution) when he has to deliver the bad news?
- From your life and professional experiences, can you give examples of how tensions have been demonstrated and managed in the breaking of bad news?

8.4   Strategies used in the delivering of bad news

In the previous two sections of this chapter we have taken a CA approach to discuss the means whereby interlocutors have managed the delivery and receipt of bad news, in that we have looked at the sequences of utterances. And we saw too in Interaction 8.1 how the conversation was co-constructed by the participants when the deliverer of news took perspectives which were different from the purely medical perspective, and this enabled us to identify a number of PDSs. By taking the patient perspective, the doctor was able to ascertain the meaning that the patient's illness had for her: its impact on her emotionally (she was 'terrified'), socially ('keeping it together', 'can't manage') and physically ('drop the baby', 'crippled with arthritis'). The patient was implicated in the conversation; this facilitated a trusting relationship such that she was able to make painful disclosures and enrich her medical history. This could inform the doctor's practice but also could allow the doctor to facilitate the aligning of the patient's perspective with the medical perspective. In Interaction 8.2 we saw how the news delivery was constructed interactionally through the four-part news delivery sequence (NDS) and how it culminated in a show of affiliation and empathy by the deliverer of bad news. In our reflections, we were able to consider how the deliverer of news aligned with the institution, and we could think more about the tensions that might arise as a result of affiliating with the recipient of news while following the institutional agenda.

Following Maynard (1996), we will now consider some further strategies which agents of bad news use in the delivery of bad news. He identifies three such strategies which we are also able to observe in our extracts of data. In Interaction 8.1, and in each of the following two situations, we might consider the news to be unwelcome, i.e. bad news. In Interaction 8.2, the supervisor is aware that the news will cause a disruption in the social order of Giovanni's life, and he appears to be considering this when approaching the topic of bad news.

8.4.1   Forecasting news

The supervisor *forecasts* the news of Giovanni's redundancy by breaking it gently, leading up to it with statements relating to the topic. Not until line 9 does his agenda become clear to Giovanni. Even at that point the news is not given directly. Rather the supervisor confirms Giovanni's *realisation* of the news (line 11), the confirmation coming in lines 13–14 ('I'm afraid I'm going to have to release you next month') when he is well into his next turn. Maynard suggests that forecasting seems to be effective in enabling the recipient's realisation of the bad news.

You can see that the discourse of the supervisor is strategic in that he is giving advance warning that the news is not good, but does not keep Giovanni in suspense. He allows him to be *co-implicated* in the event and be prepared gradually for the bad news, enabling him to come to the realisation himself of what the news will be, and the impact it will have on the social order of his life (lines 16–18). This is evidenced in the actual discourse, where you can observe the collaboration between the supervisor and Giovanni. The supervisor follows up the delivery of the news by offering some help in restoring the social order in Giovanni's life (line 15). But he goes further and demonstrates his empathy with Giovanni (lines 19–21) (see the discussion in Chapter 4 relating to empathy and affiliation). There appears to be every indication that the announcement is part of a process, and not the end of the situation. We could suggest that Giovanni's realisation of the news is a result of the quality of the relationship he has with his supervisor, and this in turn is demonstrated in the construction of their interactional discourse practices in the presentation and reception of the news.

8.4.2   Blunt news delivery

The discourse in Interaction 8.3a is a far cry from that of Interaction 8.2. In this short extract we see a disclosure of unsolicited opinion. Bad news is not given directly but in relation to a question, which is left only partially answered.

Interaction 8.3a

Claire, a 28-year-old woman with metastatic carcinoma has been referred by her oncologist to Dr A as a possible candidate for a new treatment. Her mother is accompanying Claire. She knows that Claire, more than anything, wants to be a wife and mother. After talking about the pros and cons of the regime, Dr A continues:

1 Dr A:	... so I wouldn't think of putting you on that regime
2 Claire:	(1.0) Well the other question is about getting married and whether we
3	have children or not (0.3) whether I can take the// pill
4 Dr A:	//well for someone
5	with your health problems I <u>certainly</u> wouldn't advise you to think of
6	getting pregnant right now...
7 Claire:	Oh (2.0) so now I'm <u>rea::lly</u> going to have to talk with Al

Here the doctor is seen to take a different approach to the delivery of news from that of either the doctor in Interaction 8.1 or the supervisor in Interaction 8.2. His partial response to Claire's question can only be described as *blunt*, with the result that Claire (and her mother) are left in a social vacuum. In this particular situation, Dr A goes further than giving the unwelcome news of not starting on 'the regime' and not getting pregnant. He emphasises his negative response by stressing the lexical item 'certainly' (line 5). The use of this lexical item on two occasions (line 1 and line 5) appears to emphasise his power in the interaction, giving little opportunity for questioning. Claire appears to accept this response from the doctor and then changes footing (line 7).

The risk of delivering the news/information so bluntly is that there will be *misapprehension* on the part of the recipient that could lead to her denying the situation, possibly taking it as a sick joke, not believing that anybody could be so forthright when delivering what to the recipient might well be devastating news. The disruption of the social order of Claire's life is made worse – having already had her life disrupted so many times during the trajectory of her illness – and as a result she might well allocate blame to the doctor for this further disruption. Claire must now face the prospect of telling her fiancé the news, and, in such a situation of *anomie*, the risk here is that, having received bad news so bluntly, she may have few inner resources whereby she can deliver the news to her fiancé in anything other than an equally blunt manner. A further risk of blunt inform-ings is that the chances of panic are maximised (Glaser and Strauss 1965: 143) or that the recipient will go to pieces (Glaser and Strauss 1965: 149). Maynard makes the relevant point here that 'blunt informings exacerbate the senselessness concomitant to lack of typicality, predictability, causality, and morality that bad news portends in the perceived environment' (Maynard 1996: 124).

However, there is an alternative way that this scenario may be played out (and from your experiences, you might think of other ways by which the doctor could manage the discourse.)

Interaction 8.3b

1 Dr C:	... so I wouldn't want to think of putting you on that regime without
2	you having time to consider the effects and side effects.
3 Claire:	(1.0) Hmm. Well the <u>other</u> question is about getting married and
4	whether we have children or not (0.3) whether I can take the//<u>pill</u>
5 Dr C:	// perhaps
6	this is something that we should talk about with your fiancé (..) This is
7	something that is presumably not unimportant to him (lau//ghs....)
8 Claire:	(//laughs) I should say
9 Dr C:	well what say you see the receptionist and make another appointment
10	and we could talk about your treatment and the issues of contraception

Here we see the doctor taking a very different approach to the issues raised. Although he is forthright about her treatment, he is also sensitive and offers some justification for his decision. There is, however, no blunt informing of bad news in relation to Claire's question about pregnancy and birth control. You might think that he is stalling in the delivery of news. Perhaps you believe that he is giving himself time to get to know Claire – and for Claire to build up trust in him. But it is possible that the doctor wants to ensure that Claire has the support of her fiancé in a decision that involves both of them. Importantly, perhaps he wants to ensure that her fiancé understands the seriousness of Claire's health situation. Whatever his reasons for adopting this attitude, he strategically uses discourse to lead to a closure of this interaction, but also 'keeps the door open' so that the topic can be developed when Claire returns for another appointment and she and her fiancé have talked more about their situation. This not only allows Claire to feel that she is not being 'brushed off' but, from a discourse organisational perspective, it is a strategy which allows for the construction of coherence across interactions (see Chapter 7).

8.4.3   Discourse as a focus for discussion

Interaction 8.4

Martine has recently graduated from a nursing programme and is part way through an orientation programme. She realises she does not want to continue working as a nurse but is unable to bring herself to withdraw from the programme. Her difficulties are compounded by her perception that two of the registered nurses are unhelpful and resent working with her. She has decided to talk to the Nurse Unit Manager (NUM) but does not know how to broach the topic, believing that the NUM would think she was unreliable and make it difficult for her to get other employment. She respects the NUM and does not want to create difficulties should her resignation cause staffing problems.

1 NUM:	Oh Martine come <u>in</u> how are things <u>going</u> you wanted to see me (0.3)
2	how are you settling down here
3 Martine:	Oh ehm alright I suppose (0.5)
4 NUM:	bit different from your last placement I expect
5 Martine:	Well yes it is really
6 NUM:	Yes I'm sure (0.1) you were in theatres weren't you? Rehab is quite
7	different (0.2). Here you're working so closely with the patients all the
8	time. How do you find that? (0.3) it must be quite an adjustment for you
9 Martine:	Yes well er it's quite challenging// but ehm
10 NUM:	//yes the patients have to work so hard to
11	see any impro<u>ve</u>ment and can get <u>so:</u> frustrated
12 Martine:	Yes er I've noticed that and sometimes their visitors don't appreciate
13	just how tired they get
14 NUM:	You're very perceptive for somebody who's so recently arrived here
15 Martine:	<u>Am</u> I? Do you <u>think</u> so?
16 NUM:	I <u>do</u>. I <u>also</u> hear very good things about you from the patients. You've
17	made quite an impression in a very short space of time
18 Martine:	Oh I don't know (0.2) I find it easy to talk with them (0.1) p'raps it's
19	because I'm used to talking with older people.
20 NUM:	Oh have you had a lot to do with them then?
21 Martine:	Not really just my grandparents but my grandmother had a CVA and
22	can't be hurried and her speech has been affected so we've had to be
23	very patient (.) she gets so e<u>mo</u>tional sometimes
24 NUM:	Ah that explains a <u>lot.</u> I think you have <u>so:</u>o much to give to the patients
25	and some of them have no close family or friends and will really
26	appreciate your empathetic nature. <u>Now</u> (0.5) was it the off-duty roster
27	you wanted to talk about?
28 Martine:	Partly (.05) ehm well ehm can I request some er weekend off duty ...

8.4.4   Stalling the delivery of news

Neither *forecasting* nor a *blunt* delivery of news is evident in Interaction 8.4. We see here an example of extreme *stalling*, as Martine, for whatever reason, is unable to deliver her news to the NUM. Stalling can keep the recipient in a state of indefinite suspense, as is evident when the NUM returns at the end of the extract (lines 26, 27) to the reason for the interaction. It might be suggested, however, that the NUM, as the supervisor, should bear a considerable degree of responsibility for this stalling, since the NUM takes the lead in a number of turns, making it difficult for a junior (and rather anxious) member of the team to get across her agenda easily. There is no evidence in this extract that Martine's goal of news delivery was achieved by the NUM, since it is evident in line 26 that the NUM was under a misapprehension of the reason for the meeting. There is also evidence of some collaboration here, since Martine agreed (line 28) with the NUM's opinion for the meeting, leaving Martine's actual goal unmet (i.e. announcement of her wish to leave the profession – and possibly hoping for advice from the NUM in how she might start the resignation process). We can only assume that *social psychological conditions* are present which impact on the inability of Martine to deliver her news, for example Martine's seeming embarrassment in her response line 28 ('Partly (.05) ehm well ehm can I request some er weekend off duty') and fear of loss of face (see discussion in Chapter 4) in having to admit that she has made the wrong choice of profession, and not wanting to cause workplace problems for the NUM for whom she has developed respect.

Reflective learning 8.4: Delivering bad news

There are a number of factors in each situation which appear to relate to the manner in which the news is delivered.

- Reflecting on each scenario in turn, consider the discourse strategies which indicate that the news deliverer is *forecasting* the news, being *blunt* or *stalling*.
- How, for instance, are the *turns sequentially managed* in each interaction?
- And how does the turn-taking affect the manner of news delivery?
- What markers in the discourse are indicative of the social relations between the interlocutors, and how do these relations affect the delivery of the news in each scenario?
- Now reflect on how empathy is demonstrated:
  - how is empathy demonstrated in the discourse of Giovanni's supervisor?
  - do you believe that empathy with Giovanni is a factor in the supervisor's approach to delivering the news item?
- What *critical moments* can you identify (see Chapter 7) in each of the scenarios, i.e. moments of significance which have the potential to upset the status quo?

(cont.)

Reflective learning 8.4 (cont.)

Now return to Reflective learning 8.1, but this time reflect on how you were made to feel at ease. Consider for example:

- Who delivered the news?
- What were the social relations between you, as recipient, and the deliverer of the news? How did this affect you - for example, was the news delivered by a health professional, and how long had you known each other?
- How was it delivered and what effects did this have on your realisation of the news?

8.5   Discourse strategies used in the structuring of news delivery

Much of our discussion up to this point has focused on some of the determinants of how news is given and the impact this has on the social order. What we need to consider now is how the conversations are structured in what are frequently difficult encounters. We already noted the turn-taking sequences in the situations outlined above and identified through them a gradual unfolding of facts, or lead-in, to the announcement of bad news, as in Interactions 8.1 and 8.3 (cf. Glaser and Strauss 1965).

We saw how the conversations in each of the three Interactions were *co-constructed*, with no one person exclusively holding the floor – turns were given and taken with few interruptions. In their paper: 'Bad news in oncology: How physician and patient talk about death and dying without using those words', Lutfey and Maynard (1998) found that the disclosure of bad news was inter-actionally structured. When we examine the structure of the interaction between Giovanni and the supervisor, we find that the discourse is strategic in that neither Giovanni nor the supervisor refers directly to the source of the bad news – 'retrenchment', 'being laid off', 'being dismissed', albeit for different reasons. The supervisor was forecasting the news and breaking it gently. Giovanni, however, even when he came to the point of realisation, did not mention the word 'retrenchment', but immediately talked about its effects – the rupture in his social life. The event was framed in terms of a PDS, the interaction being organised to co-implicate the recipient's perspective. The sequence allows the deliverer of news to give news carefully and gently, 'teasing out' the interlocutor's opinion, so that the news is gradually unpackaged. It is a tool which allows the realisation of the news and enables the recipient to adapt to the situation.

Interaction 8.5

Mr Davis is re-telling the event of his wife's sudden death after she'd left home to go to the women's mid-week service in the local chapel.

Oh dear (sigh1.0) I was just making a cuppa <u>tea</u> and there was a knock on the <u>door</u>. It was Jack <u>Edge</u> from the police. (2.0) Oh ... this is <u>too</u> hard. (1.0) I <u>thought</u> maybe he was looking for <u>Huw our son</u> he's always in demand (0.2) so <u>busy</u> with people wanting him to sort out their <u>problems</u>. He was looking so <u>serious</u>. I er asked him <u>in</u> and if he wanted a <u>cup</u>. He <u>didn't</u> but I was about to warm the <u>teapot</u> and (0.5) oh <u>dear</u> (0.5). He <u>said</u> (.05) '<u>look</u> let's go and sit <u>down</u> Bern'. He was looking <u>really</u> con<u>cern</u>ed We knew each other from the <u>rugby</u> see. 'No no' I said 'we can talk <u>here</u> while I'm making the <u>tea</u> (.3) but <u>you</u> sit down'. And em he said 'No I think we ought to have a talk sitting <u>down</u>'. Well he was looking very <u>serious</u>, not a <u>glimmer</u> of a <u>smile</u>. And that's un<u>u</u>sual for him because he's <u>always</u> up for a laugh (0.2). I wondered <u>then</u> if anything was the <u>matter</u>. But why didn't he <u>ring</u> me from the <u>station</u>? Oh I don't <u>know</u> (0.5)(<i>sigh</i>) Huw was at <u>work</u> and Jane's living up <u>north</u>. I <u>wondered</u> maybe one of the <u>children</u> was ill but then why didn't she <u>ring</u> me? It <u>still</u> didn't click. 'Well if you in<u>sist</u>' I said and sat <u>down</u> here in the kitchen with him. He was <u>fiddling</u> with his hat and I noticed he seemed to turn his phone off. I think that <u>must</u> have been his own mobile so I asked him if something was the <u>matter</u>? 'Well er I'm af<u>raid</u> the news isn't <u>good</u> em (0.5) Bern when did you last see Mrs Davis?' So I <u>told</u> him ''bout an <u>hour</u> ago (0.2) she'll <u>be back</u> after the women's service if you want to <u>talk</u> to her'. 'No no I want to talk to <u>you</u>' he said 'I'm afraid it's <u>about</u> Mrs Davis. (0.5) Was she al<u>right</u> (0.2) when she left here?' So I thought she'd been taken <u>ill</u> and he wanted to take me to where she <u>was</u>. By <u>this</u> time I wasn't <u>thinking</u> straight. Well you <u>ca:n't</u> can you Oh de:<u>ar</u> (0.5) (<i>sigh</i>) and then he <u>told</u> me (0.2) e:<u>ver</u> so con<u>side</u>rate he was that she'd col<u>lapsed</u> in the town centre, and there was a <u>police</u>woman near who tried to re<u>sus</u>citate her but it was no <u>good</u> and (0.2) o:h what a to do (2.0) <u>Huw</u> was in work and <u>Jane</u> (2.0) oh <u>dear</u> this is <u>too</u> much. You <u>know</u> he spent an <u>hour</u> with me I don't know <u>what</u> I'd have done with<u>out</u> him (1.0) he sent for my <u>son</u> and even <u>stayed</u> with me til <u>Huw</u> got ho:me...

Reflective learning 8.5: Non-verbal communication

> Following our discussion and analysis of the earlier four Interactions, you now have the opportunity to analyse the situation in Interaction 8.5, where bad news is given not by a healthcare practitioner, but by a police officer who has been deputed to break the news of the death of a 73-year-old woman to her husband. The family is well known and highly regarded in the community, being active in many community events and activities.
>
> (cont.)

Reflective learning 8.5 (cont.)

Consider the following points

- While we have made only passing reference to non-verbal aspects of communication, they are an essential component of our communication strategies. From your acquired knowledge from everyday experiences and professional practice, can you identify some of the aspects of this narrative where non-verbal communication is of extreme importance?
- What is significant about the place of the interaction and the position in the community of the interlocutors in this situation?
- How did the police officer handle the spatial aspects of the interaction?
- How might the officer respond to Mr Davis's tears, sighs and pauses?
- How have *you* responded to Mr Davis's sighs and pauses?
- From this narrative, what strategies of the police officer can you detect that he used in the delivery of news? For example, can you identify an NDS or PDS? Was the news forecast given bluntly or was the news stalled? What discourse feature can you identify in the breaking of news?
- How might the officer identify Mr Davis's needs?
- Reflect on a situation where you might have to inform a person of the death of a loved one. How do you think you might handle the situation? (As well as the discourse, consider, for example, the spatial, temporal and cultural aspects.)

What is important to acknowledge, and is exemplified in this extract of Mr Davis's narrative, is that words, and therefore discourse, can never tell the 'whole story'. There are many questions we need to ask if we are to empathise with Mr Davis's situation (see Chapter 4), not least of them being the type of relationship which Mr and Mrs Davis had developed over the years. Other factors of significance must be considered, such as the duration of their marriage, the presence of family and friends, the support network and relationships.

However, we must be wary of giving our own interpretations to situations, particularly if we are not directly involved in the situation. For instance, we are reminded that discourse analysts must analyse the discourse and leave the interpretation of the total situation to others who are professionally qualified to do so. Such an approach encourages a multidimensional approach to discourse practice and can result in an enhanced understanding of the discourse. It has the potential to enrich professional relationships between colleagues from different disciplines and have an emancipatory and liberating effect on the individual practitioner.

8.6   Summary

In this chapter, we have discussed the complexities involved in delivering bad news, and have found that in most instances the disclosure of bad news does not 'just happen'. The discourse is interactionally structured and strategic to ensure that the desired outcomes in difficult situations are achieved. The difficulties confronted by the deliverer of bad news are highlighted when these outcomes have not been achieved, exemplified in a situation where the delivery is stalled (see Interaction 8.4). We are left wondering whether there has been a misunderstanding between the interlocutors about the purpose of the encounter. Did a seemingly sensitive interlocutor, who was the professionally more senior partner, in fact simply fail to engage in sensitive listening? Or did the initiator of the interaction fail to present a clear proposition? Similarly, we might question whether the doctor who delivered news bluntly understood the impact of a traumatic situation on his interlocutor (see Interaction 8.4). Or did the interlocutor, for whatever reason, present her questions in such a matter of fact manner that the doctor responded in a seemingly equally matter of fact manner, i.e. *mirroring* his interlocutor's behaviour? Was the doctor insensitive? Was the patient attempting to save face (see the discussion in Chapter 4)? How else might the interaction have developed?

In contrast to these discourse situations of miscommunication, we considered the effectiveness on the recipient of news when the news was forecast by the deliverer, such that news was unfolded gradually and delivered with sensitivity (Interaction 8.2). By focusing on a device which Maynard identifies as the perspective display series (PDS), we were able to frame the analysis of yet another situation. By co-implicating the patient's perspectives (Interaction 8.1) and involving her in the interaction, we were able to discuss the effects of this strategic use of discourse on the local outcomes of news delivery. These questions, as we have posed them, refer only to the verbal aspects of the interactions, and so we concluded our activities with the narrative account of a person who had received bad news. From this we were able to consider just some of the non-verbal aspects of discourse, complementing the 'what was said' with 'what was not said': the silences, pauses, sighs, kinesics. As well, we considered the identity of the deliverer of news and significant others in the event. The question that remains to be answered now is the adequacy of our analysis of the interactions. Can we ever consider events in isolation without being cognisant of extraneous factors? What we have emphasised throughout the discussion in this chapter, and indeed throughout the book, is the importance of the wider situation – the healthcare situation and the culture – and the meaning that this gives to the event and to the local situation. The demands of the discourse situations such as we have presented in this chapter are challenging for the healthcare practitioner and require skills which are not of necessity easily achieved. But as we have seen in this, and preceding chapters, the discourse of practitioners is such that they must necessarily function at a high level of communicative expertise. In Chapter 9 we will observe how healthcare practitioners achieve the level of expert in their discourse practices and discuss how the construction of coherent discourse is one of the markers of expertise.

Further reading

Maynard, D. (2003). *Bad news, good news: Conversational order in everyday talk and clinical settings*. Chicago: University of Chicago Press.

9 The Expert Practitioner: Professional Expertise and Communicative Expertise

Concepts to be introduced, explored and applied

- The 'expert' practitioner
- Professional expertise versus communicative expertise
- Markers of the expert discourse practitioner
- Coherence in discourse

Objectives of this chapter
After completing the study of this chapter you will be able to:

- understand the concept of communicative expertise in professional practice;
- analyse the discourse of the expert practitioner, discussing it as a contributing factor to expert professional practice;
- consider levels of communicative expertise in workplace discourse by comparing the discourse of the expert practitioner with that of a novice;
- identify coherence as a key aspect of professional communication and the discourse factors which contribute to its production.

9.1   Introduction

This chapter, together with Chapter 11, will address the nature of expertise and, in line with our concerns in this book, specifically focus on communicative expertise. We will be drawing upon and utilising concepts addressed in previous chapters to inform our discussion. When we reflect on our professional practice, or observe the practice of others, we recognise that our practice changes with experience as we learn to adapt to different situations to which we are exposed. We argue that continued exposure to situations which demand specific skills results in improved skills performance, and often results in changes to the approaches we take to performing tasks. While initially we are conscious of protocols and guidelines to be followed to perform a task, and the steps taken to complete it, with exposure we perform the task 'automatically', knowing exactly what needs to be done – and how to do it. In a familiar situation we home in on the exact nature of the demands placed upon us, barely thinking about the process required to achieve positive results. Schön (1983) asserted that competent practitioners usually know more than they say, demonstrating their tacit knowledge. Of interest is that he believed that practitioners often seemed able to reflect on their intuitive knowledge – their knowing-in-action – and when they were in the process of action they were able to use this when situations were uncertain and conflicted.

9.2   Developing expertise

Benner (1984), building upon the work of Dreyfus and Dreyfus (1980) and Dreyfus (1982), presented insights into the process by which we achieve such expertise. Interestingly, where the focus of the study of Dreyfus and Dreyfus was upon airline pilots and chess players, that of Benner was upon nurses. She demonstrated that, whatever our workplace, expertise is skill specific and develops gradually with exposure to experience. Our position here is that communication is just such a complex skill and is also situation specific. However, just because we are skilled at communicating with friends in everyday situations, this does not, and should not, imply that we are skilled when communicating with patients and indeed with our colleagues in all environments. When we consider the World of Communication (S. Candlin 1992, 2008) discussed in Chapter 1, we proposed there that our discourse is dependent upon our awareness of certain variables ('sensitivities'), and as such, we should not be surprised if our performance in response to the demands of different situations might also be equally variable. To explore this, we again analyse the discourse of health professionals in a discourse-based health activity to identify factors which contribute to the development of what we believe is just one of the markers of communicative expertise, namely creating/constructing a coherent discourse event and, importantly, determining the effects on discourse outcomes as they relate to healthcare. Here we should make the point that we are referring to *coherence* as being mainly concerned with the features which connect topics and thus maintain topical coherence, for example the overlapping in an interaction of two lexical items which, in the minds of the interlocutors are both connected with a topic; see the example from Interaction 9.1 (below). 'Rubber mat' and 'my stick' are lexical items which can be seen to be features of creating a safe environment.

16 Jane:	and the rubber mat now that you've //got
17 Mrs C:	//my stick has been

Related to our discussion is the notion of adherence to rules; Wittgenstein (1958) proposed that conversations can be regarded as a collection of language games which, like all games, are defined by rules. Constraints (as well as opportunities) therefore are placed on speakers, and so successful accomplishment of the goals of conversation depends upon cooperation between the participants. 'Playing the game' demands that each player (speaker) not only plays by the rules, but also acknowledges that conversations, like games, have goals where those of speakers may or may not be in accord with those of their interlocutors. Moreover, in the case of healthcare communication, we need to consider as well as the goals of the patient and carer, those of the institution. In sum, a *coherent* conversation is one where the interlocutors' contributions bear some sort of relationship to a goal, and where connectedness between each other's contributions plays a central role.

Reflective learning 9.1: Language games

Reflect on the notion of language games. From your everyday experience, do you believe that there are ('folklore') rules about who can say what to whom in healthcare settings?

- Consider some of the 'rules' about who can say what to whom? For example, what can a doctor or a nurse say to patient but a patient would not say to the health carer?
- How do you think these beliefs about behaviours relate to the situation in your workplace?
- Do you agree that the interactions of patients and health carers can be likened to this idea of 'language games'? Would you say that your answer is confirmed by the evidence we have seen in the interactions you have studied in this book (including Interaction 9.1 below)?

9.2.1   Discourse as a focus for discussion

In our analysis of the extracts of data, you will see that coherence in the discourse is not just a matter of obeying rules, but reflects the cooperative element in successful communication. It demands an awareness of the means whereby interlocutors co-construct their discourse. This in turn reflects how clearly the event is framed (see Chapter 3), but it also demands on the part of the participants:

- sensitive listening,
- attention to non-verbal signals (evidence which, of course, is not always available to us, as we analyse in this book just the verbal discourse),
- the production of sequential turns (see Chapter 2),
- topic management (see Chapter 2),
- acknowledgement of past, and sometimes shared, history,
- utilising both tacit and newly acquired knowledge.

In working through this process, you will come to appreciate the hybrid nature of your discourse and the production of what we may call *interdiscursive* text (see the discussion in Chapter 6).

Interaction 9.1

Jane RN delivering nursing care to Mrs C at home in the community.

2 Jane:	… we're just going to be talking about you (…) and how you are	
3	how you manage at home that sort of thing. We've been coming	
4	to you for some months now haven't we?	
5 Mrs C:	yes=	
6 Jane:	=helping you with your showering. You're starting to feel better	
7	about that <u>now</u> aren't you	
8 Mrs C:	oh yes feeling more confident too	
9 Jane:	mm that's good	
10 Mrs C:	but as I say you know if I didn't feel well and I was (?)	
11	I wouldn't have=	
12 Jane:	=that's right you're better off not to on	
13	those odd days and you're sure there's a nice support	
14	in that shower with the rail and all that in it	
15 Mrs C:	yes=	
16 Jane:	=and the rubber mat now that you've //got	
17 Mrs C:	//my stick has been	
18	in the kitchen for two days not used=	
19 Jane:	=right so you're	
20	becoming stronger//that's good// isn't it	
21 Mrs C:	//yes I nearly//had a little slip in the	
22	bathroom last night. I tell you what I did in the bathroom	
23	one //night// before I go to bed	
Jane	// mm //	
24 Mrs C:	I might go to bed about half past five or something like that	
25	but I put the light on in the bathroom all night and the first	

26		time I turn it off is when I get up in the morn//ing //
27 Jane:		//that//'s a good
28		idea isn't it just gives a bit of light around
29 Mrs C:		yes and it gives me a little bit of con//fidence//
30 Jane:		//that's right//

Interaction 9.2

175 Mrs C:	and then of course I've got me back brush too
176	when I get a littler more confidence I can use that
177 Jane:	well that's good isn't it
178 Mrs C:	I don't em in the wintertime I only use a brush on m back about
179	once a week which is enough because you're not [?]
180 Jane:	well your skin's pretty good isn't it
Mrs C:	mm
181 Jane:	well that's what we'll do we'll just keep going *a* tiny bit
182	longer until you're absolutely confident that you can
183	manage yourself but it's great to think you're wanting to
184	have a go now. It's a//start//
185 Mrs C:	//yes I // was telling my sister
186	yesterday and she said don't get too confident
187 Jane:	no well there's no point in //that too//
188 Mrs C:	//she said// she said you are on the verge
189	I am on the verge like I do have a lot of falls (..) I pulled that door
190	down one night just (?*)//you know//
191 Jane:	//yeah yeah//

Reflective learning 9.2: Revisiting Chapters 2 and 3

When analysing the discourse in Interactions 9.1 and 9.2, reflect on your learning in Chapters 2 and 3 and think for example about:
- the indications in the discourse that Mrs C understands what the interaction is all about and how it will proceed
- how the interactions are framed

- Do you consider that the framing has made it possible for Jane to achieve both her discoursal and her nursing goals?

(cont.)

Reflective learning 9.2 (cont.)

- What strategies do the interlocutors use which demonstrate a free-flowing interaction, the 'content' of which is pertinent to the frame set by the nurse and tacitly agreed to by the patient, and how is this tacit agreement demonstrated?

Reflective learning 9.3: Co-construction of the interaction

In the extracts of data you will notice that some words recur.

- Draw a line which links those words. Do you notice a recurring theme carried by the words in question? If so, who initiated this theme, and why is the identity of this person significant?
- How is Mrs C's tacit agreement demonstrated in the discourse?
- How was cooperation in the discourse demonstrated? For example, what discourse features can you identify suggesting that the interlocutors cooperate to encourage continuation of the theme?
- What features can you identify which suggest that the interaction is co-constructed between the interlocutors?[1]

9.2.2 Analysing the discourse

We can make a number of observations when we consider the way that discourse strategies are utilised, such that they become key factors in the structure of the interaction. For example, in Interactions 9.1 and 9.2 you will probably have observed that Interaction 9.1 is framed as a talk about the patient: how Mrs C manages at home and 'that sort of thing'.

Jane accommodates to Mrs C's knowledge base, avoiding the professional (and more formal) term 'assessment', which might not be one with which Mrs C is familiar in this context. Mrs C's tacit agreement to participate in such an interaction is seen by her positive response (line 5) and then her volunteering of an extended answer in line 8.

The discourse is seen to be co-constructed by the nurse and patient, with Jane using more casual terms (e.g. the metaphors (see Chapter 8) 'nice support' (line 13), 'just keep going', 'tiny bit' (line 13)), creating an atmosphere of informality and allowing their turns to overlap.

Turns are taken sequentially: questions are asked and answers given which are

---

[1] See the Appendix at the end of this chapter. Do you agree with our observations?

often extended so that the following turns provide more information or a change in footing, e.g. lines 17 and 20 (see discussion in Chapter 3).

In your analysis you may have identified 'confidence' as a lexical item that recurs throughout these two extracts, suggesting that it is of concern to Mrs C. Jane demonstrates that she is actively listening to her interlocutor (see the back channelling in lines 9 and 23 – 'mm') and also, after making pertinent comments throughout the exchanges, she demonstrates to Mrs C, in line 182, that 'confidence' – which Mrs C initiated – is a key issue in her decision-making and is related to the continuation of her care. Although a number of topics in the data are discussed, there is a relatedness between many of them; for example, we might say that 'safety' is an underlying feature in lines 12–22, where support, rail, rubber mat and stick are mentioned. This is confirmed when Mrs C talks about 'nearly having a little slip in the bathroom'.

However she then appears to change footing by talking about putting on the light, and while Jane appears to make the connection to 'safety', Mrs C returns to the theme of 'confidence' in line 29. The whole effect of the interaction is one which is coherent. Coherence involves, for example, topic management and turn-taking and also conversational relatedness, which in turn is related to consistency, relevancy and order, features which are demonstrated in the discourse of the interlocutors.

9.3   Strategies for developing coherence in the discourse

This might be a good moment to think about how our observations and analysis are reflected in the research literature, turning to the work of Kendon (1992) to illuminate our discussion. Kendon's point is that where two or more participants interact there is a joint transaction between the interlocutors such that there is a tacit agreement about the way in which the interaction is conducted. This is unique for them in that moment of time and is different from other interactions. There is order in the transaction and a definition of roles: 'If the co-participants are willing to follow the participant's lead, they will make complementary moves ... and so maintain the status quo' (Kendon 1992: 331). Kendon implies that successful actions, of which discourse is a central part, is a cooperative venture, strategically executed and co-constructed by the participants. This co-construction contributes in no small part to the development of coherent discourse – an interaction that is free-flowing in its delivery and consistent in its application to the subject matter. Coherence demands smooth turn-taking (see Chapter 2), which in turn involves sensitivity to the other person's needs. Drawing upon the work of Ribeiro (1996), Tannen (1984) and Goffman (1974), we can say that coherence is also closely linked to the ways in which a discourse event is framed. It is in the framing of the discourse that the scene is set. The interlocutors need to understand what the event is about and how it will be conducted, i.e. what the 'rules' are that govern the conduct, for example the degree of formality or informality, the topics which are permissible or not permissible, and whether the topics can recur. Attending to these features, and others, determines how the conversation will flow.

Goffman (1974) writes about the *story line* and the *attentional tracks* which help direct this flow of conversation, something which we see in the data where the term 'confidence' occurs a number of times. 'Confidence' appears in line 26 (in relation to the safety of the light) as the beginning of what we might suggest is a theme. Later in the conversation, in line 182, confidence is raised again and relates to time; and in line 186 it relates to the topic of social support (line 185). In line 190 the topic of social support relates to that of safety (line 189). Both participants are co-constructing this conversation with the nurse evidencing her listening skills in her responses and overlapping utterances (lines 24, 27, 187, 191). This clearly supports Kendon's position when he talks of *complementary* moves. Our argument here ties in closely with Goffman's (1981) notion of attentional tracks. He proposes that in any social encounter there is an activity which moves the event further along. This activity is within the *main-line* or *story-line track*, and is relevant to the successful understanding of the event by both participants. Our argument is that this is a prerequisite of cooperative discourse and at the same time also relates to the construction of a coherent discourse.

Let us now take a look at the theme of confidence as being just one such attentional track.

Reflective learning 9.4: Attentional tracks

Consider again the interaction of Mrs C and Jane. To guide your reflections, consider the following:

- Can you identify any themes other than *confidence* in their discourse?
- If so do you consider these additional themes strengthen the coherence of the interaction?

Now reflect upon a recent conversation you have had with a patient, colleague or friend that you consider was coherent.

- Identify themes in it that contribute to its coherence
- How does that conversation contrast with one that you consider lacked such coherence?

Chafe (1992) offers another useful perspective in this search for coherence. He talks about ideas in discourse being in an *active* state or a *semi-active* state. We can see from the two brief extracts of data above that themes are discussed and appear again in future utterances – in such instances we might suggest that the topic, e.g, the topic of *confidence*, forms a strand. Although the idea of strands acting as *directional tracks* helps to establish coherence in the discourse, this does not explain why topics (e.g. related to confidence) appear and re-appear without upsetting the coherence of the interaction. Topics must of course be motivationally relevant to that point in the discourse – that is, relevant not only to the speaker but to the interlocutor. We make assumptions that both speakers will remember and understand the nature of the reference to a previously raised topic or track. Chafe (1992) suggests that there is a limit to the person's cognitive capacity and sooner or later *active ideas*, that is topics within the discourse, must lose their active status, making room for new ideas. He argues that ideas do not immediately become *inactive* when not being talked about, but enter a state of *semi-activity*. He states,

> [R]oughly speaking this [*semi-activity*] is a state that functions as a holding area for ideas that may later be re-activated as they re-enter the discourse. It is also a state within which separately activated ideas are conceptually integrated into a larger picture. Semi-activation presumably has a great deal to do with the preserving of coherence within a discourse. While ideas are in a semi-active state they are accessible and can be re-activated and re-enter the discourse … (Chafe 1992: 270).

We could argue that this process allows for coherence across a number of interactions over time, making sense to the participants – but not necessarily to those observers who have not shared the discourse history (see Chapter 11). In our extracts of data (Interactions 9.1 and 9.2 above) we might say that the coherence in the discourse is also dependent upon Jane's tacit knowledge and her professional judgement. However, if we make this proposition we will have to question the nature of what we mean by professional judgement. Some might argue that such judgement is intuitive and tacit but, as we noted from our discussion of the expert practitioner, this apparent intuitiveness and tacit knowledge is built upon a wealth of experience and in-depth knowledge. Such experience of course relies not just on practice experience, but on a sound educational base. Bordage (1994) argues that professional judgement also requires drawing on sets of criteria in evaluating options, and makes the particular point that, while criteria can be taught, they are useless until the student accumulates a substantial amount of experience by applying such criteria in a wide variety of unstructured situations. If practice at applying the criteria is absent, the criteria remain merely abstractions. We can see this exercise of professional judgement and intuitive knowledge in the discourse of the expert practitioner.

9.3.1   Discourse as a focus for discussion

Interaction 9.3

125	Jane:	yeah you look nice and strong on your legs
126	Mrs C:	anyhow I go (/)
127	Jane:	It's a while since you've been out isn't it?
128	Mrs C:	yeah I haven't been out what do you mean out of the house?
129	Jane:	Outside yeah
130	Mrs C:	I haven't been out at all
131	Jane:	No but you're going to want to go out aren't you?
132	Mrs C:	Yeah
134	Jane:	We talked a bit that extended day care but you didn't seem
135		interested in that are you// not
136	Mrs C:	//no I've got too many friends that I can't keep
137		up with them
138	Jane:	Yeah and they pop in and you play a good game of cards I hear don't you

Interaction 9.4

379	Mrs C:	Now I haven't been I haven't seen the butcher since March He'll wonder
380		where I am unless somebody's (.) I don't know and the lady who has the
381		little shop unless (..) you know the little (?) shop
382	Jane:	It's only close isn't it but you've got that little hill
383	Mrs C:	yes and I think I'll take the stick out
384	Jane:	Oh I would
385	Mrs C:	I've got that sti//ck
386	Jane:	//don't venture out without your stick

Reflective learning 9.5: Coherence

Consider the Interactions 9.3 and 9.4 above, keeping in mind our discussions related to constructing a coherent discourse. To guide your reflections:

- Trace any topics which run through the discourse of the participants. How do they constitute themes which occur and re-occur as suggested by Chafe (1992)?
- Is one participant more active in maintaining coherence in the discourses, and does this pattern change across the extract?

(cont.)

Reflective learning 9.5 (cont.)

- Comment on this: for example, is one person in control of the topic and if so, what does this tell you about the power relations between the interlocutors?
- From your own professional experiences, can you give examples when conversations were coherent or not coherent? What differences can you identify in the discourses that inform your opinions?
- Reflect now on the coherence of the discourses of Jane and Mrs C and Sara and Mrs Y in Chapter 7 (Interactions 7.3 and 7.4). From your reading and helped by the discussions in this book, as well as reflecting on your professional experiences, can you suggest any factors which contribute to the coherence of the discourses?

Interaction 9.5

Now examine the brief extract of data below between a care assistant and a resident in an aged care facility

167 Naomi:	...physical assessment em you're bed bound now aren't you?
168 Mrs B:	yes
169 Naomi:	(..) no outdoor ability have you?
170 Mrs B:	No
171 Naomi:	None
172 Mrs B:	Unfortunately
173 Naomi:	er your lower limbs well they're em (...)
174 Mrs B:	Well I have all this bowel trouble but I don't now what to name it (.)
175	but it worries more than anything
176 Naomi:	mm inability. Your activities of daily living ...

Reflective learning 9.6: Framing and topic management

- What features in the discourse can you identify that indicate the approach which Naomi takes to the activity? For example, would you say that this is framed as a conversation? Who appears to be dominant in the interaction?

(cont.)

Reflective learning 9.6 (cont.)

- What are the indicators that you consider make for a coherent interaction in Chafe's sense? Is there a return to topics for example?
- Can you account for any differences in the manner in which this interaction is conducted compared with those of Jane and Mrs C in interactions 9.1, 9.2, 9.3 and 9.4?

9.4   Comparing the discourse of the expert practitioner with that of the novice practitioner

While Naomi follows the procedure of assessment in accordance with the instructions as she has understood them, perhaps her discourse is indeed coherent but only at a local level. She is following a series of items on a proforma without deviating from it, as we can see when she disallows a change of topic attempted by Mrs B (line 176). By not acknowledging Mrs B's contribution Naomi is not displaying appropriate listening skills, and there is no sense that the interaction is being co-constructed by the interlocutors. Naomi's discourse strategies are quite different from those of Jane in her interaction with Mrs C. There we see Jane allowing expansions of topics; drawing upon her knowledge of Mrs C, she ensures that topics are motivationally relevant to Mrs C and also to Jane as she fulfils her professional and discoursal goals. For example, mobility and the use of aids – such as a walking stick and rails in the bathroom – is of relevance to Mrs C because they concern her safety and ability to perform activities of daily living, such as shopping and walking in areas that are demanding. But mobility is relevant too to her social needs such as 'wanting to go out'. For Jane, the relevance of mobility is also related to improvement in health (Interaction 9.4, line 125).

While we might say that there is an element of coherence in each of the nurse–patient conversations, we could also make the point that the coherence demonstrated by Jane and Mrs C is more comprehensive than that demonstrated by Naomi and Mrs B. We might suggest that the coherence of their discourse is simple coherence in that there is little extension of turns, and the information requested by Naomi is not made relevant to Mrs B's situation. Jane's obvious sense of the relevance of the information provided by Mrs C to Mrs C's overall health situation and needs, as well as Jane's ability to reinforce and make relevant to Mrs C the information obtained in the conversation, is evidence, we would argue, that Jane is an expert practitioner. She immediately homes in on Mrs C's situation and by expanding on known and new information guarantees that its relevance is understood by Mrs C. See, for example, line 127 where she begins the topic related to social health and everyday life: 'It's a while since you've been out isn't it?' Similarly in line 386 ('don't venture out without your stick') she implicitly refers to the topic of safety discussed in Interaction 9. 1.

Jane learns about Mrs C's specific needs in the interaction and is able to revise her professional goals. She listens and co-constructs the interaction with her interlocutor, blending the discourse genres of the social world of Mrs C with those of the professional world of healthcare. This is evident, for example, in line 138 when she says, 'Yeah and they pop in and you play a good game of cards I hear don't you?' in response to Mrs C's mention of the important topic of her friends. Jane's expertise lies in her ability to maintain social roles and purposes of both herself and Mrs C. Her actions are purposive and intended to achieve ends. It is this which contributes to the overall notion of coherence, providing a very firm connection between coherence in interactions and expertise in practice, where the aims of the institution are achieved. We can note a link between Jane's expertise, her professional judgement and tacit knowledge, since she is experienced in performing this professional practice of eliciting relevant information on which her care is based. Her care demands a sound knowledge of health needs, goal identification and the interventions necessary to meet health needs and goals. This knowledge in turn is augmented by observational skills and, particularly, discourse skills which facilitate the disclosure of information pertinent to the situation. Such disclosure can be face-threatening and demands sensitivity to the patient's perceptions – only achievable by the use of appropriate discourse, both verbal and non-verbal.

9.5   Summary

In this chapter we have considered the concept of expert discourse practice suggesting that discourse coherence is a criterion indicative of the expert discourse practitioner. At the same time, we do need to acknowledge that practitioners in the healthcare workplace (or, indeed, any other workplace) whose expertise is revealed through their discourse are not necessarily expert clinical practitioners. In the same way, practitioners whose clinical skills demonstrate expertise may not necessarily display expert discourse skills. Experts in one situation are not necessarily experts in other situations. What we can say, though, is that discoursal expertise enhances clinical practice, when professionally that practice is already at the level of the expert.

Building on the discussion in this and previous chapters, consider the communication strategies that contribute to achieving coherent discourse. We could suggest the following strategies are also salient in the achievement of coherent discourse:

- observing non-verbal signs (for example: gestures, facial expressions, use of space – see, e.g., Chapter 1 and the World of Communication);

- utilising attentive listening skills;
- facilitating smooth topic control by using strategies to initiate, maintain, expand and/or change topics when appropriate (see, e.g., Chapter 2);
- identifying triggers, e.g. lexical items, to 'change footing' (and topics) to create a new frame (see, e.g., Chapter 3);
- reintroducing and reusing topics as appropriate so that a theme is formed that runs through the text but,
- acknowledging that there may be more than one theme in the discourse – demanding an ability to keep 'more than one ball in the air' at a time (as discussed in this chapter);
- taking advantage of a shared history where topics can be raised appropriately from previous encounters (see, e.g., Chapter 11).

Now that we have at our disposal a useful toolbox of communication strategies to help us understand the principles of communication in healthcare practice, in the next chapter we will reflect on situations where communication within the multidisciplinary team is a focal point. This will necessarily involve discussing the notion of the community of practice and its impact on the identities of the individual, as well as the person's roles and responsibilities.

Appendix 9.1

(See Reflective learning 9.3)
Some features identified in the analysis of the discourse of Jane and Mrs C.

- Note the links between the underlying theme of confidence demonstrated by underlining.
- References to 'time' are indicated by italics, to 'safety' in bold, and to 'social support' in bold italics.

Reflective learning activity 9.1

2 Jane:	... we're just going to be talking about you (...) and how you are
3	how you manage at home that sort of thing. We've been coming
4	to you for *some months* now haven't we?
5 Mrs C:	yes=
6 Jane:	=helping you with your showering. You're starting to feel better
7	about that *now* aren't you
8 Mrs C:	oh yes feeling more <u>confident</u> too
9 Jane:	mm that's good
10 Mrs C:	but as I say you know if I didn't feel well and I was (?)
11	I wouldn't have=
12 Jane:	=that's right you're better off not to on

13		those *odd days* and you're sure there's a **nice support**
14		in that shower with the **rail** and all that in it
15	Mrs C:	yes=
16	Jane:	=and the **rubber mat** now that you've //got
17	Mrs C:	//**my stick** has been
18		in the kitchen for *two days* not used=
19	Jane:	=right so you're
20		becoming stronger//that's good// isn't it
21	Mrs C:	//yes I nearly//had a **little slip** in the
22		bathroom *last night*. I tell you what I did in the bathroom
23		one //night// *before* I go to bed
	Jane	// mm //
24	Mrs C:	I might go to bed about *half past five* or something like that
25		but I put the light on in the bathroom *all night* and the first
26		time I turn it off is when I get up in the *morn//ing* //
27	Jane:	//that//'s a good
28		idea isn't it just gives a bit of light around
29	Mrs C:	yes and it gives me a little bit of con//fidence//
30	Jane:	//that's right//

Reflective learning activity 9.2

175	Mrs C:	and then of course I've got me back brush too
176		when I get a littler more confidence I can use that
177	Jane:	well that's good isn't it
178	Mrs C:	I don't em on the *wintertime* I only use a brush on m back about
179		*once a week* which is enough because you're not [?]
180	Jane:	well you're skin's pretty good isn't it
	Mrs C:	mm
181	Jane:	well that's what we'll do we'll just keep going *a tiny bit*
182		*longer* until you're absolutely confident that you can
183		manage yourself but it's great to think you're wanting to
184		have a go *now*. It's a//start//
185	Mrs C:	//yes I // was telling **my sister**
186		*yesterday* and **she** said don't get too confident
187	Jane:	no well there's no point in //that too//
188	Mrs C:	//**she** said// **she** said you are on the verge
189		I am on the verge like I do have a lot of falls (..) I pulled that door
190		down *one night* just (?*)//you know//

10   Communication in Healthcare Teams

Concepts to be introduced, explored and applied

- Community of practice (CoP)
- Competing and conflicting roles and responsibilities
- Role identities

Objectives of this chapter
After completing the study of this chapter you will be able to:

- understand the concept of 'community of practice';
- examine possible changes in identity as a result of membership of the CoP;
- consider the multidisciplinary team as one such CoP;
- discuss the roles and responsibilities of team members as a discourse community.

10.1   Introduction

There is increasing scrutiny by the general public and researchers across academic disciplines, specifically those in health communication studies, of the work and organisation of hospital based healthcare. The resulting discussions are well exemplified in the book edited by Rick Iedema (2007), *The discourse of hospital communication: Tracing complexities in contemporary health care organizations*. The research reported in that book, for example, by Lum and Fitzgerald (2007), Kerosuo (2007), Barton (2007) and others, discusses the complexity of discourse relationships in the dynamics of hospital organisations, and contextualises clinical-professional discourse. As one example, Castells (1990) argues that contemporary workplaces are increasingly being reconfigured into becoming knowledge/information/communication networks demanding 'not just more knowledge and information, but more intelligent and affective practices generally' (Iedema 2007: 6); 'employees have to be able to negotiate difference and dissent among one another and "organizationalize" their feelings, relations and selves' (Iedema and Scheeres 2003). Drawing upon the work of Pincock (2004) and Sutcliffe, Lewton, and Rosenthal (2004), Iedema highlights how:

> the emphasis on 'situated communication and clinical interaction' … derived from the now widely shared acknowledgement that the quality of communications and interactions among the clinicians is to a large extent a determiner of the outcomes of their work for patients. The efficacy of what clinicians do for patients – the ultimate protagonists in health care – depends of course in an important way on clinicians' expert-professional acumen. However it is also increasingly clear that achieving good clinical outcomes for patients is contingent on interprofessional and professional–patient communication about the systemization and dynamic co-ordination of care processes (Iedema 2007: 2).

In the same way, Weick and Sutcliffe (2001, cited in Iedema 2007: 2) draw our attention to the need for mutual expectations and relationships over the substance of care. For some, this could be seen as a departure from traditional medically dominated practices and representative of change in the delivery of care. Change, then, may include an increasing focus on multidisciplinary care teams; while many welcome this development, such change can become a site of tensions, as professionals' knowledge and understanding of the work of others may be called into question. Iedema argues that 'clinicians have no choice but to re-think their professional–occupational relationship, their power balances and their self-identities' (2007: 6). Such tensions and subsequent resolutions are to be worked out in the discourse of colleagues as we show in the illustrations below.

Illustration 10.1

| Community Nurse: | I visited Mrs Smith today and noticed she had no handrail on the stairs. Would it be possible to install one? |
| Occupational Therapist: | I'll assess the patient and decide whether she needs a handrail. |

Illustration 10.2

On a later occasion, the same nurse said:

> …Improving practice means understanding what other professional colleagues do which then also helps us to become effective members of a multi-disciplinary team. Thankfully

healthcare is more team-based these days, both in terms of nursing teams and multi-disciplinary teams. And as someone who has worked in a multi-disciplinary team I know how enriching the experience can be. I learned so much from other team members.

(data extract: Candlin and Candlin 2007)

While we can detect the tensions that are apparent in the newly formed team in Illustration 10.1, the nurse, reflecting on her experiences, recognised that communication was a major factor in what might result in a breakdown in professional relationships. She addressed this apparent deficit in her communication, and, as can be see in Illustration 10.2, she later regarded her work experience very positively.

In the context of discussing such communication in teams and teamwork, Candlin and Candlin (2007), drawing upon the earlier work of Lave and Wenger (1991) and Wenger (1998), turn to their concept of a *community of practice* (CoP) when they discuss the impact of multidisciplinary teams on both role identity and relationships within such teams. Reporting on research gathered from conversations with nurses from different specialty areas of practice reflecting on their experience, they found not only changing patterns in the structure of teams, but also how change had brought about the development of different, and more egalitarian teams. One participant said,

I learned so much from being part of a team: from the aged care nurses, physios, OTs, speech therapists, dieticians, social workers, geriatricians. It took a while to break down the barriers created by territorial ownership of specialties. But once we got to know people and relate to them we learned so much from each other and we developed a healthy respect for each other. I often felt I had more in common with team members from different professions than I did with members of my own profession.

(data extract, Candlin and Candlin 2007)

In effect, this nurse was identifying herself not just as a member of her professional body, but as a member of a CoP located in aged care, and specifically being identified as an aged care nurse.

Reflective learning 10.1: Ascribed identities

Reflect on your professional life and experiences.

- How do you think you are identified? How has your identity seem to have changed over the duration of your working life?

(cont.)

Reflective learning 10.1 (cont.)

Now think about your social life outside of the work setting.

- How do you think you are identified in the various contexts and activities in which you engage as a participant?

10.1.1 Discourse as a focus of discussion

Interaction 10.1

(Note that this interaction was first discussed in Chapter 1.)

The multidisciplinary team in the Department of Aged Care at St James Hospital is meeting for its weekly case conference. The team consists of the consultant geriatrician (Dr Tony Diaz), registrar (Dr David Bowen), nurse consultant (Jenny Fogerty), physiotherapist (Anne McEnroe), occupational therapist (Jodie Curnow) and speech pathologist (Elisabeth Carter). They are discussing the care of Mr Delaney, who was admitted during the night via the Emergency Department, presenting with a history of headache, slurring of speech and weakness of the left side.

1 Consultant:	We've now come to the new patients. David you were on call last
2	night. Tell us about Mr Delaney.
3 Registrar:	Yes, well Mr Delaney came in early this morning. He's 68, a recently
4	retired financial planner, previously well apart from a history of
5	hypertension. He fell when he got up to go to the bathroom last night
6	and his wife noticed some oddities in his speech. Fortunately she
7	called an ambulance and they brought him straight here. He had a BP
8	reading of 180/90 on arrival, with a left hemiparesis, dysarthria and
9	what looked like an expressive dysphasia as well. The CT in
10	Emergency showed no haemorrhage, so he had intravenous tPA as
11	per the protocol. He's been on anti-hypertensives for a number of
12	years, but by all accounts was otherwise healthy.
13 Consultant:	OK so what investigations have you ordered?
14 Registrar:	Ah.. an MRI, chest x-ray, blood profile an//d//
15 Consultant:	//OK//. Don't suppose
16	anybody else has seen him apart from the nurses. Jenny what can you add?
17 Nurse consultant:	Well he's feeling pretty sick and confused at the moment. He's not
18	eaten much, his swallowing's not good, he's nauseous, incontinent, takes
19	two to lift. His left arm's oedematous and all up he's not a well man.
20 Consultant:	Hmm lot of work ahead here. I'll see him after the conference and then
21	I want to talk with his wife. Anne you'll be doing an assessment today

22	won't you?
23 Physiotherapist:	Yes. I want to see how soon we can check his balance so we can plan
24	his program.
25 Speech pathologist:	Yes and I want to know what his swallowing reflex is like, see if we
26	need nasogastric feeding. I'd like to see Mrs Delaney too, she must be
27	pretty distressed about his speech. See how soon we can get her
28	working with us.
30 Consultant:	Right, who's next Jenny? How's Mrs Smith doing?

Interaction 10.2

Following the weekly case conference, the consultant (Tony Diaz) and nurse consultant (Jenny Fogerty) are waiting to talk with Mrs Delaney.

1 Nurse consultant:	Mrs Delaney must be worried out of her mind and to make matters
2	worse, she's an RN. They've both just retired and were planning 'the
3	big trip'
4 Consultant:	Yes she's probably upset about travel plans.
5 Nurse consultant:	Oh it's not just that. She's feeling guilty because she says her husband
6	had a brief episode of 'odd speech' last week but they didn't take it
7	seriously. Now she thinks the excitement over the cruise has triggered
8	it off.
9 Consultant:	Hmm I can imagine, but at least as a nurse she'll understand what we're
10	doing.
11 Nurse consultant:	Let's hope so but I don't know what area she's worked in. She was so
12	worried about her husband and telling the family and didn't say much
13	about herself.
14 Consultant:	Ah here she is. Mrs Delaney do come in, take a seat. I'm Tony Diaz,
15	the consultant geriatrician and of course you've met Jenny, our nurse
16	consultant. I expect you're rather worried aren't you? This must have
17	been quite a shock for you
18 Mrs Delaney:	You're not wrong there. Thank goodness I've got the family nearby.
19 Consultant:	Yes I expect that's a comfort. Jenny tells me you were planning a big
20	trip. That must be a disappointment,
21 Mrs Delaney:	Oh I don't care about that. I'm more worried about Jack
22 Consultant:	I imagine. How much do you understand about Mr Delaney's situation?
23 Mrs Delaney:	Not a lot. I know I'm a nurse//but
24 Consultant:	//oh you are? *(feigning surprise)*
25 Mrs Delaney:	Yes but its years since I worked anywhere other than Child Health
26 Consultant:	You'll probably see some changes but we'll tell you what we're doing

27		and why. We start the rehab program as soon as we can.
28	Mrs Delaney:	Really, so soon? How long will he be bedfast then?
29	Consultant:	Once he's been seen by Anne, she's our physio- we'll know how soon
30		we can start getting him mobile. Then he'll be seen by Jodie, the OT,
31		and the speech pathologist, Elisabeth – well I should say you'll both be
32		seen by them because I expect you'll want to be involved in his//rehab
33	Mrs Delaney:	//oh I
34		don't know much about this, I've been with Mums and Bubs for a//ges
35	Nurse consultant:	//no
36		but you'll have a head start on most of our carers. And we'll be working
37		with you all the way – after all you'll be his chief support and we all
38		work as a team here, Mr Delaney, when his headache's lifted, you, and
39		everybody here
40	Mrs Delaney:	I'm so worried. Do you honestly think he'll recover OK? I don't want
41		him in an aged care facility.
42	Consultant:	Look we're talking a little way down the track. Let's take it a 'step at a
43		time'
44		There's a lot of work for everybody but first we'll have to see about
45		some tests, scans and things so we know exactly what's going on.

Reflective learning 10.2: Discourse in clinical practice

Drawing upon your reflections when you were first presented with the above scenarios in Chapter 1 (Section 1.4), and following on from your further learning experiences, can you now identify issues of communication in the discourse? For example, and to guide your reflections:

- What can you say about the control of topics and the management of turns in the interactions? Who, in fact, appears to control the interaction?
- What comments can you make about how overlapping speech and interruptions are managed? What are the effects of these features, and their management, on the outcomes of the discourse?
- How might the interaction be conducted differently?

10.1.2   Commentary on the data and the reflection activity

When you study the discourse of members of the multidisciplinary team (Inter-action 10.1), you might consider that topics are raised within a team setting and are dealt with immediately, sometimes in only one or two utterances. Look, for example, at line 23 when the physiotherapist responds to the consultant's comment by providing information about her plan for rehabilitation for the patient.

Illustration 10.3

21 (Consultant)	... Anne you'll be doing an assessment today
22	won't you?
23 Physiotherapist:	Yes. I want to see how soon we can check his balance so we can plan
24	his program.
25 Speech pathologist:	Yes and I want to know what his swallowing reflex is like, see if we
26	need ...

Immediately, the speech pathologist gives an unsolicited comment about her plans for assessment. Neither comment elicits further discussion; each utterance seems to have become *inactive* and is not raised again in the interaction (see the discussion in Chapter 9 and the work of Chafe). These topic areas become part of the history of an interaction and – in the case conference situation – contribute to an understanding by team members of the patient's history. The discussion contributes to a pool of knowledge to be reactivated by team members, and as such becomes not only an event of a particular moment and shared by those present, but part of a body of knowledge. It can also be used as appropriate, and within the bounds of ethical considerations (such as confidentiality, beneficence and non-maleficence), by other team members who care for the patient. What this means is that discussion in such instances, informs and becomes part of future discussions. The contents of topics discussed are seen never to completely decay but are retained, not only in individual memories, but often in written mode, for example in notes taken at the time, which then constitute part of the patient's medical history. Interactions in conferences then take on an essential temporal dimension, occurring at a given point in time, but also to be reactivated later for therapy purposes or as points of comparison to monitor progress. In Chapter 3 we discussed the notion of topic control and in Chapter 9, drawing on the work of Chafe, we acknowledged how topic control and sequential turns contributed to discourse coherence. In this chapter we can extend the discussion further and see the practical application of this theory in the delivery of healthcare. But we can also suggest tentatively that coherence can transcend the boundaries of a single speech event, since ideas can be developed in later interactions.

Reflective learning 10.3: Coherence revisited and the reactivation of ideas

Reflect on the quotation from Chafe 1992: 270 (above, p. 136) and with reference to the interactions in this chapter.

- What evidence can you find in the discourse for ideas being reactivated?
- What examples can you find in the discourse to suggest that there is (or is not) coherence across speech events, i.e. the two interactions?
- Reflecting on your professional experiences, how would you say that these extracts of discourse in a team represent your professional practices in the clinical setting?
- What safeguards are in place that ensure that interactions between colleagues, patients and team members, and patient's family and team members, conform to ethical standards in your workplace?

10.2   Community of practice

You are now in a position to think further about the practices of the multidisciplinary team and consider whether you believe that the team is an example of a community of practice (CoP) referred to earlier. The construct of the CoP was first developed by Lave and Wenger (1991) and Wenger (1998), and has since been used extensively across a range of disciplines. But as we will see in our discussion, the construct of late has come under some challenge in the healthcare field, for example by Candlin and Candlin (2007).

Eckert and McConnell-Ginet describe the CoP in the following terms:

> an aggregate of people who come together around mutual engagement in an endeavour. Ways of doing things, ways of talking, beliefs, values, power relations – in short practices – emerge in the course of this mutual endeavour. As a social construct, a community of practice is different from the traditional community, primarily because it is defined simultaneously by its membership and by the practice in which that membership engages (Eckert and McConnell-Ginet 1992: 464).

What is interesting about this definition is the way it emphasises the *raison d'être* of the community as gathering around mutual engagement in an endeavour. This in turn suggests a goal orientation of the group, a point taken up by Scollon, who defines a community of practice as 'a group of people who over a period of time share some set of social practices geared towards some common purpose.

Everyone is multiply membered in various communities of practice' (Scollon 1998: 13). This definition of the CoP as a community of multiple memberships allows us to recognize how the members of such a group can be continually enriched by the various other CoPs. At the same time, we need to acknowledge that there will always be the potential for tensions to arise as issues of members' competing priorities and agendas influence the dynamics of the community. We can detect this in the earlier interaction in this chapter between a community nurse and an occupational therapist (see Section 10.1, Illustration 10.2).

Reflective learning 10.4: The notion of CoP

Consider the interaction between the occupational therapist and the community nurse in Interaction 10.2 above.

- What factors in the discourse indicate that this is a functioning multidisciplinary team who form a CoP in the manner described by Eckert and McConnell-Ginet (1992) and Scollon (1998)?
- How does your membership of a CoP (whether or not you work in a multidisciplinary team) in your workplace differ from your membership of a social group such as your family? Think in terms of the criteria suggested in the description given by Eckert and McConnell-Ginet. How does their description differ from Scollon's definition?
- What effects do you think membership of a CoP might have on interprofessional relationships, and how do these relationships affect patient outcomes (for example, see the illustration earlier in this chapter between a community nurse and an occupational therapist, and compare that with the discourse of the multidisciplinary team above)?
- In your opinion, how does the formation of CoPs affect discourse practices, professional practice and professional development?
- What alternative practice of care delivery have you experienced?

The complexity of any CoP suggests that there has to be some necessary governance and regulation for it to be effective and indeed for it to develop. Sarangi and Roberts (1999: 16) make the key point that 'The institutional order [of a *community of practice*] is held together not by particular forms of social organisation but by regulating discourses' (Sarangi and Roberts 1999: 16). We could even say that the institutional order *is* dependent upon the social organisation, in that such an organisation has been created and maintained by strategically utilised discourse. We might even suggest that the emergence of CoPs is, for many workplaces, part of the New Work Order described by Iedema and Scheeres (2003), where employees are increasingly required to negotiate differences and points of dissent among one another, and 'organisationalise' their feelings, relations and selves. In effect, they need to be skilled not only at developing professional relationships, but at team building, acknowledging each other's professional skills and also the complementarity of such skills. This in turn requires acknowledging and understanding the roles and functions of each other, calling for appreciation not only of self-identity, but of the identity of others. This acknowledgement was provided by an intensive care nurse when she said:

> We also work within a multi-disciplinary team, and value the contributions of social workers and other allied health professionals

> (data extract Candlin and Candlin 2007: 253)

Discussion of such multidisciplinarity serves to concretise the concept of CoP working together to address situations and problems. Perhaps you can find evidence in the discourses above of how members of the team worked together to address situations and problems. These communities are not isolated units but work together in a situation of mutual concern, their practices overlapping (Figure 10.1). Within members of different professional groups (i.e. other CoPs), health outcomes and personal growth can be enhanced as the 'spaces' occupied by individuals overlap with those of others. The extent of this overlap has, of course, to be negotiated, recognised and respected if the utility of the team's strengths and contributions is to be maximised for the benefit of patient outcomes and team cohesion.

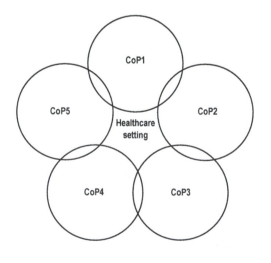

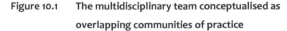

Figure 10.1   The multidisciplinary team conceptualised as
overlapping communities of practice

But this sharing of space where multidisciplinary teams represent the New Work Order can be challenging and also unsettling, as Iedema and Scheeres go on to note and discuss:

> First they affect most workplace participants, leaving few untouched: members of management, workers and professionals. Second the ways in which individuals respond to these changes vary. For some, building new relationships, learning new practices, changing allegiances, and shifting work focus can be unsettling and even debilitating: for others it can be empowering and offer opportunities (Iedema and Scheeres 2003: 319).

The positive effects of 'empowering and offer[ing] opportunities' as a result of working within multidisciplinary teams has been the experience of Sue (trained in the 1970s) working in the area of nuclear medicine. She feels valued as the nurse in the team and is often consulted on issues related to nursing:

> As the only nurse on the team, I am often approached for my opinion. I feel valued

This confirmed her previous experiences working in aged care in the early 1990s, as did the experience of the community nurse in Illustrations 10.1 and 10.2 in this chapter. While Sue's experience was positive from the start, and even empowering, the community nurse had to work through an indifferent beginning which made considerable demands on her attention to relationship building and the strategic use of discourse. Only after much working through issues related to communication issues was the nurse able to view her experience positively. CoPs are made up of members who are multiply membered (see Scollon 1998) in that they are members of different CoPs. But within a specific CoP, their practices may overlap those of other members as is exemplified in Figure 10.2. For example, the physiotherapist is a member of her professional body – the CoP of physiotherapists, but at the same time is a member of the CoP of aged care specialists. (The members exemplified here might of course also involve other members of CoPs such as social workers).

To understand the contribution which members of the CoP can make, each member needs to be aware of the skills of others. These skills can be represented not just by the expectations of the professional body or members of the public, but through the behaviours and practices each member might perform at a given time, depending upon the situation and individual need (see Figure 10.3). Practices often overlap and are represented not just by different discourses of the nurse's voices as she speaks with the voice of the counsellor, the healer/carer or the advocate, or on other occasions where we might hear the voice of the researcher or the manager. In each situation she might adopt a different identity realised not only by physical actions, but by particular discourses. The nurse manager may be in a meeting with other managers from different disciplines,

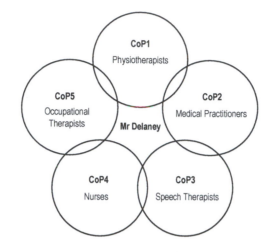

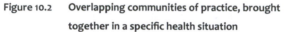

Figure 10.2   **Overlapping communities of practice, brought together in a specific health situation**

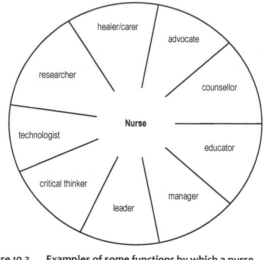

Figure 10.3   **Examples of some functions by which a nurse might be identified at any given time**

listening to presentations or making a presentation, negotiating for resources, advocating for the CoP of nursing. In another situation she may be engaged in discussion with (nursing) team members about staffing issues and allocation of resources at a local/ward level. And so we see that not only is the CoP multiply membered, but so too each member adopts multiple *identities*. Central to the person's professional identity is that of the nurse. A nurse who is identified in a particular situation as a counsellor or an educator might also exhibit features of a healer/carer and/or an advocate. Similarly, a nurse who is identified as a technologist might also be engaging in practices associated with those of a researcher and/ or a healer/carer. As the profession continues to evolve through advances in technology, sociopolitical-cultural change, educational opportunities and (often) changes in societal and individual values and beliefs, it is likely that these underlying identities and practices will also change.

Reflective learning 10.5: Professional identities

Reflect on the situation in your workplace.

- How are you identified in different professional practice situations?
- Who identifies you as such: e.g. self, patients, colleagues from your own profession, colleagues from other professions?
- How do you believe these identities are enacted in your discourse, by your behaviours?
- How are these identities a reflection of your education, life/professional experiences, culture, values, beliefs?
- What are the core values, beliefs and behaviours which are shared amongst different health disciplines?
- How do these commonalities represent a unifying force such that it impacts on the identity and ethos of the team?

10.2.1   The extent of 'mutuality of engagement'

We have discussed some of the practices and identities of the nurse as an example of the work of one member of the CoP, the nurse, but we have also reflected on our own individual practice and behaviours. However, as Eckert and McConnell-Ginet (1992: 462) indicate, a CoP is an 'aggregate of people who come together around mutual engagement in an endeavour' and they go on to make the point that 'Ways of doing things, ways of talking, beliefs, values, power relations – in short practices – emerge in the course of this mutual endeavour'. What this suggests is that members are engaged in cooperative work, where they are in tune one with another, and although they are not performing similar behaviours, each member works in ways so that the practice of one impacts upon and enhances the practices of another, jointly aimed at achieving optimal patient outcomes. This depth of teamwork reminds us of the work of Hak (1999), who, when observing two nurses caring for different patients in an ICU environment, noted that one, without either of them appearing to say anything or to signal to the other, stopped what she was doing and went to the aid of the other. This is not an unusual occurrence when nurses work together in the same specialty area, and as one ICU nurse remarked when hearing about it said, 'Well of course, we're doing it all the time'. She seemed to be implying that ICU nurses are confronted by situations everyday and are in tune with each other. Situations are mutually understood and resources are utilised appropriately.

Reflective learning 10.6: Tacit knowledge

Within a CoP, defined either by profession or by a particular medical specialty, can you identify instances where verbal communication was unnecessary for a task to be accomplished successfully?

- Reflecting on an example of such a situation, can you identify any factors which contributed to a mutual understanding of the situational needs?
  - Were actions determined by knowledge and understanding of the context: patient needs, treatment and caring protocols, etc?
  - To what extent were the professional personal relationships determining factors in your behaviour?
  - To what extent was education and experience underpinning factors in your responses?
  - Do you believe that the responsive behaviour such as that observed by Hak can be taught?
- Would such immediate responses be possible for a person who was new to a specific workplace?

Reflective learning 10.7: Mutuality of engagement

- When considering the work of Hak, and from your own experiences, how do you consider that behaviours such as those observed by Hak suggest the existence of a 'mutuality of engagement' and a 'joint enterprise' with members having mutual goals?

Reflect on the scenarios in this chapter in light of the discussions that we have engaged in throughout this book.

- What patterns in the discourse can you identify which indicate that members of the CoP are mutually engaged, that they have mutual goals and that they are engaging in a joint enterprise?
- Do you think that your membership of the CoP of a multidisciplinary team would identify you more as a member of that CoP rather than 'your own' professional CoP?

When we reflect on the previous activity, and in particular on the final question, it is worth considering that a few practitioners feel they have more in common with the other workers in the team than they do with members of their own profession. In contrast, there are those who think differently, who are identified first and foremost as a member of their own profession, not only by themselves, but by other team members who recognise their special expertise on which others can draw. In this way, they can be said to enhance the CoP of the 'workplace' and contribute positively to patient outcomes without, however, denying their unique professional identity. They are multiply membered and possess multiple identities.

10.3   Summary

In this chapter we have referred to the New Work Order (Iedema and Scheeres 2003) and drawn on the concept of the community of practice (Lave and Wenger 1991; Wenger 1998). We have explored and illustrated the structure and workings of a CoP through our example of a multidisciplinary team working in an aged care setting as one such community. We have also identified some of the complexities associated with the workings of such a team in terms of the multiple identities of team members, and we have emphasised the role of discourse in the achievement of social and professional goals. Candlin and Candlin (2007) highlight this problematic area when they write, 'given professional training and expertise, and enabled by enhanced interpersonal communication skills, practitioners can manage this multiplicity through negotiation and consensus building ...', and when they conclude:

> [C]ommunities are bound, individually and together, not by the institutions of medicine, nursing, or the bureaucracy, but by altruistic caring, and the desire to meet human needs. This meeting of need is mediated by the compassionate caring of health professionals and by developing and engaging in a high level of discourse competence ... (Candlin and Candlin 2007: 264).

In Chapter 11, we will discuss how power and trust are established within the healthcare team, or the community of practice, and the impact that ethical dilemmas have for its members.

Further reading

Candlin, S. (2011). Changes in professional identity: Nursing roles and practices. In C. Candlin and S. Sarangi (eds.), *Handbook of communication in organisations and professions*. Handbook of applied linguistics, 3. Berlin: Mouton de Gruyter: 551-69.

11   Healthcare Teams: Leadership, Power and Ethical Dilemmas

Concepts to be introduced, explored and applied

* Leadership
* Power
* Ethical dilemmas and consensus building

Objectives of this chapter
After completing the study of this chapter you will be able to:

* identify different styles/types of leadership and the discourse features that characterise them;
* describe some of the differences between a 'leader' and a 'manager' and work out how these two concepts might be distinguished;
* understand some of the ways in which 'power' can shape interactions;
* analyse the discourse features of consensus building in healthcare teams, focusing especially on ethical dilemmas and the processes by which they are 'worked through'.

11.1   Introduction

In this chapter, we will begin by looking at ways in which 'leadership' is performed through our use of discourse, and discuss some of the distinctions that are often made between 'leaders' and 'managers'. We will then bring the notion of 'power' into the equation, focusing once again on how the power that individuals hold influences the way that they manage professional interactions. This engages us with a discussion of ethical dilemmas, so that we can highlight ways in which members of healthcare teams (or communities of practice) work through such dilemmas. The process of coming to grips with ethical dilemmas illustrates the importance of understanding the discourse of consensus building, and how power and leadership are inevitably involved in that process.

11.2   Leadership

People have looked at leadership from a wide range of perspectives. Our focus here is on the ways in which we can understand leadership as a 'discourse practice' in healthcare settings. How do people enact their leadership roles through the language that they use in interacting with others? In this section, we begin by conceptualising 'leaders' as those who hold officially designated leadership positions, as well as those who assume the role unofficially or are looked upon as a leader by others.

Holmes, Schnurr, Chan and Chiles (2003) suggest that the concept of leadership embodies two main elements. The first of these is what they call the *transactional* component, which includes the issues at hand to be attended to, as well as the outcomes to be achieved. The second is a *relational* component, which involves attention to interpersonal relationships between the leader and members of the team. Although effective leadership can be thought of narrowly in terms of measurable outcomes, for us 'leadership' implies the involvement of more than one person, highlighting the essential relational aspects of leadership. We focus here on those 'processes' – particularly the discourse processes involved in performing various styles of leadership.

Reflective Learning 11.1: Leaders and managers

Recall our earlier discussion of communities of practice (CoP) in Chapter 10. What sorts of teams or CoPs exist in your workplace? For instance, a small private practice may consist essentially of a single CoP, while a large hospital may consist of many CoPs, with individuals belonging to more than one.

- Who leads these teams? How is this leadership formally designated (e.g. this is sometimes done through an official title such as head, director, CEO, chair, supervisor, team leader). Is the leadership fixed, or does it rotate regularly between members?
- What are the relationships between the leader(s) and other members of these teams (e.g. professional colleagues, teacher-student, etc.)?
- Do you see yourself as a 'leader' of any of the CoPs to which you belong?

(cont.)

Reflective Learning 11.1 (cont.)

- Do you see a clear distinction between a 'leader' and a 'manager', or do you see these terms as overlapping in meaning?

Personal experience tells us that there is no single style of leadership. The way in which people approach the task of leading others varies enormously according to their individual styles as well as the *culture* in which they are operating. Following Tannen (1989), we can think of 'culture' as a multilevel concept. On one level, we have the mainstream culture of the society at large, which may be relatively homogeneous or nowadays, with migration, increasingly heterogeneous. At another level we can talk about the culture of the broad types of organisation or institution (business culture, academic culture, healthcare culture, for instance). Looking more closely, we can identify the culture of the institution concerned (e.g. that of a particular hospital). Finally, each individual CoP within a particular organisation will have its own local culture, implying that styles of leadership may vary greatly even from one 'team' to another. The 'relational' aspects of leadership make it necessary for leaders to address the face wants (see our discussion in Chapter 4) of those whom they are leading. The cultural constraints (and affordances) that are in play at the many levels we outline above will determine the expectations that people have about the way in which their face wants are respected (or not!). What is seen as appropriate and constructive behaviour in terms of building good relationships in one context may be completely out of place in another.

11.2.1   Discourse as a focus for discussion

Interaction 11.1

Liz is a specialist in emergency medicine, and is conducting a clinical tutorial for two medical students, May and Rob.

1 Liz:	OK so you're the resident, May, and you've just seen this
2	patient (.) what are you going to do?
3 May:	well, I'd do an MRI urgently, and-
4 Liz:	do an MRI? You mean you'd wheel in the machine and set it up
5	[*general laughter*]
6 May:	[*laughs*] uh no sorry (.) I'd be calling the consultant on-call first
7	and giving them the history
8 Liz:	Right, OK, great (.) now it's 2 AM and Dr Kim's on call, you all

9	know Dr Kim? Very approachable and friendly, won't mind being
10	woken up at 2 AM (.) what'll you tell her?
11 May:	Well she won't have seen this patient before so I think I need
12	to fill her in on the background history first, and then explain
13	you know that the patient has suddenly become ah (.) drowsy
14	and disoriented, and um I'm concerned that there might have
15	been further bleeding, and that's why I want to get an MRI (.)
16	if she agrees of course
17 Liz:	OK good (.) um, now the thing to remember is when you talk to
18	the person on-call you want to show that you've thought about the
19	situation and that you can um (.) arrange the information in a
20	meaningful way (.) rather than just going through a rigid kind of
21	checklist or pro-forma
22 Rob:	so like can we use the structure that we practised for our exams last
23	year ah (.) for presenting cases I mean, or
24 Liz:	well that's a good basic framework but you have to (.) I mean, what
25	you can try to work on now is tailoring it to different situations, so like
26	if it's a leisurely lunchtime clinical case presentation it's OK to keep
27	the audience guessing, but if it's a real-life medical emergency that's
28	unfolding, we need to um (.) prioritise somewhat, right?

Reflective learning 11.2: Leadership and facework

Consider the interaction between Liz and her students in Interaction 11.1.

- What features of the discourse do you think indicate that Liz is the 'leader' in this context?
- What seem to be the purely 'transactional' elements of this encounter?
- How does Liz attend to the 'face wants' of the group members in this encounter?
- Do you consider any of Liz's responses to be potentially face-threatening? How (if at all) does Liz mitigate these potential face threats?
- What do you think of Liz's use of humour in this encounter? How might that influence the impression that she projects to the students present? Can you see any risks associated with the use of this sort of humour as a leader?

Interaction 11.2

David is the senior physiotherapist on a neurological rehabilitation unit, and also holds the formal position of Director of Physiotherapy Services. Samuel is a fully qualified physiotherapist who graduated only a year ago, and he has just started work on this particular unit. He asks David to check a discharge note that he has just written for one of the patients in the unit.

1 Samuel:	Ah David, I've written um (.) Dr West asked me to write a	
2	discharge note for Mrs Williams because she's going	
3	home today	
4 David:	right	
5 Samuel:	and well I've done it but could you maybe have a look to	
6	see if it's what you'd normally //write//	
7 David:		//sure//
8 Samuel:	'cos it's not something I've done before (.) where I	
9	worked the doctors just wrote one discharge summary	
10	and that was all (..) it's here [*points to the note that he has written*]	
11 David:	[*reads*] yeah (.) it's basically (.) I mean you've got most of	
12	the essential points there um (.) what we usually try to do	
13	is give a <u>bit</u> more information to the outpatient physio	
14	about exactly what we've been doing //so that//	
15 Samuel:		//doing (.)// OK
16 David:	like they can just pick up from there and hopefully they	
17	don't need to call us to ask	
18 Samuel:	I see (.) sure	
19 David:	so if you could just maybe um (.) summarise her current	
20	treatment in a bit more detail that'd be great	
21 Samuel:	OK (.) will do (.) thanks for that	
22 David:	no worries at all (.) look, it's basically fine, that's really all	
23	I'd suggest	

Reflective learning 11.3: Approaches to leadership

Looking back at interactions 11.1 and 11.2:

- How does David perform the leadership role, from a discourse perspective? What specific features (covered earlier in this book) do you think are salient in the way that he provides advice to his junior colleague?

(cont.)

Reflective learning 11.3 (cont.)

- How does David's approach contrast with that of Liz in the previous scenario? What factors might account for the differences?
- If David approached his leader's role here in a similar manner to the approach that Liz adopted with May and Rob, what kinds of relational outcomes could you envisage?
- Is David performing primarily the role of a 'manager' or a 'leader' here?

Interactions 11.1 and 11.2 present two contrasting leadership styles, suited to two different leadership contexts. Liz's style illustrates what could be called 'teaching leadership' while David's style is rather what one could label 'collegial leadership'. From an 'interactional management' perspective, Liz takes a much more controlling role in (for instance) setting the topic, allocating turns, and interrupting to correct and offer commentary and advice. She uses some positive face strategies to make the students 'feel good'. For example, she places one of them in a 'junior doctor' role for the purposes of the exercise and (in lines 10 and 17) gives brief but positive appraisals of this student's performance. A more risky approach is evident when she interrupts May to make a joke of her opening words (line 4); this is a potentially face-threatening move, as it could make May feel foolish in front of her fellow student. The fact that she laughs (with the others) and moves quickly to correct her opening suggests that she does not take it this way, however. The fact that Liz then moves quickly to praise May's reformulated answer also helps to mitigate any potential face threat. Towards the end of the interaction, Liz again employs humour in making her point, but this time the joke is made without 'targeting' anything that either student has said.

David's style (in Interaction 11.2) is very different. Samuel has asked for his advice, but in carrying out his leadership role he does not appear to adopt the role of a didactic teacher. Samuel seems quite tentative in his initial request, perhaps feeling slightly awkward that (as a fully qualified physiotherapist) he is asking another member of the profession to check his work. David appears to handle the professional relationship sensitively and carefully in offering advice. He uses strategies such as *hedging* ('if you could just maybe summarise her treatment in a bit more detail …', lines 18–19) and *indirectness* ('what we usually try to do is …', line 11, rather than 'what you need to do is …') to soften the suggestions, and to avoid threatening Samuel's negative face (i.e. his 'want' to be in control of the actions he takes). In this way, David shows respect for Samuel's status as a full member of the profession, and as someone who will be able to decide how to make changes to the final discharge note. Finally, David points out at several junctures that what Samuel has written looks 'basically fine'.

Is David a leader or a manager here? Some commentators have pointed out that leaders have 'followers' while managers have 'subordinates'. As David's formally designated position of authority makes him Samuel's supervisor, he could certainly be seen as a manager here. However, if Samuel truly values his advice and follows it not merely because he feels that he ought to do so, he (David) could be seen as embodying some of the qualities of a leader as well. While leaders are often said to be people with 'vision' and are therefore focused on the outcomes or products that their leadership can facilitate, managers are characterised as being more concerned with overseeing the processes that are followed. From this perspective, David seems to be acting very much in the role of a manager. Does this mean, then, that he cannot at the same time be a leader for his team?

In a now classic article, Zaleznik (1992) argued that leaders tend to have very different personality traits from those who seek out (and are best suited to) managerial roles. While managers are problem-solvers who generally favour rationality and control, leaders (according to Zaleznik) are often temperamentally disposed to take high risks if they can see great potential rewards from the outcomes that may follow. This characterisation suggests that it might be difficult for one person to be both an effective leader and an effective manager. For Bennis (1999), there is also a fundamental difference:

> There is a profound difference between management and leadership, and both are important. To manage means to bring about, to accomplish, to have charge of or responsibility for, to conduct. Leading is influencing, guiding in a direction, course, action, opinion. The distinction is crucial (Bennis 1999: 9).

When we look at Bennis's descriptions of what 'management' and 'leadership' entail, we can say that many senior positions in the field of healthcare ideally involve skills covering both concepts. However, while we may be able to draw sharp distinctions conceptually between 'leaders/leadership', and 'managers/management', it becomes much more difficult in practice to draw such sharp distinctions when we examine the roles people actually play in their professional lives.

At this point, you may like to reflect again on your answer to the final question in Reflective learning 11.3. In light of our discussion, how (if at all) has your view changed on whether David is performing a 'leadership' or 'management' role here?

11.3   Power

So far in this book we have analysed interactions involving participants of 'unequal' status. This inequality naturally raises concerns about the presence and significance of power in professional relationships. In this section, we will look at ways in which power can be *displayed* through discourse, as well as ways in which discourses can serve as ways of *maintaining* or reinforcing existing power structures of hierarchies. As power is central to the concept of leadership, we will also revisit Interactions 11.1 and 11.2 in this section of the chapter.

Power is at once everywhere to be found but difficult to define. As the French writer Foucault pointed out, power is like a *capillary network*, running like blood throughout the system. One way of narrowing it down is to focus, as we do in this book, on communication and professional relationships, and for that we need a system for describing different types of power based on relational criteria. Such a system, proposed by French and Raven (1959) more than fifty years ago, is still relevant and used today to explore power structures in institutions. They identified what they called five bases of power. To these they came to add a sixth form of power (informational influence), one which is very applicable to power relationships in healthcare settings, and so we include it below.

1. *Positional power* (also known as legitimate power). This is the formal authority that an individual holds because of the position that the individual occupies within an organisation. It is often accompanied by 'markers' of power, such as a uniform (e.g. in the military), a large and well-appointed office (e.g. in a company, hospital or university). This is the most visible form of power in an organisation.

2. *Referent power.* This refers to the ability of individuals with particular personal attributes (sometimes known as 'charisma') to attract and influence others. These specific personal attributes or traits attract the admiration of others who wish to identify with them, thus creating the opportunity for influence.

3. *Expert power.* This form of power is grounded in the particular expertise (which may include skills and/or knowledge) that an individual has, and is proportionate to the need that others (individuals, groups or organisations) have for this particular expertise.

4. *Reward power.* Reward power stems from an ability to confer rewards that are valued by others. These may include 'material' rewards such as financial benefits or promotions, or other sorts of rewards such as praise or positive evaluation. The positive exercising of such power can lead to workplace relationships where people feel valued by others, while the negative exercise (or even abuse) of such power can lead to resentment and allegations of favouritism.

5. *Coercive power.* As we noted in Chapter 5, persuading someone to do something involves convincing them that a particular course of action is helpful in realising a goal that they have for themselves. Coercion, on the other hand, involves using your authority to influence a person to take a particular course of action because you want them to, and at the same time raising the likelihood of negative consequences if they do not. Thus power has the capacity to produce such negative consequences. At the same time, while coercive power is generally cast in negative terms, it may be wielded unwittingly in some cases, as indi-

viduals may not be consciously aware that their position means that people may feel coerced by them (when in fact no coercion was intended). Or people may do what you want them to do *without* your exercising coercive power at all, in other words they *collude* with your potential exercise of power.

6. *Informational influence*. If one person (or group) has access to information that others want or need, this creates a power relationship between them. In situations where the information-holder is seen to be withholding it (in part or entirely) from someone who feels that they are entitled to share this information, resentment or even anger is likely to result. Recent advances in information technology mean that more and more 'information' is becoming openly accessible. However, privileged information about individuals (e.g. results of medical investigations, examinations and workplace performance appraisals) remains one domain where people must seek access to information through those who hold it.

Fairclough suggests that power in discourse involves 'powerful participants controlling and constraining the contributions of non-powerful participants' (1989: 46). These controls and constraints, according to Fairclough, can operate at three basic levels:

1. *Contents*: the sorts of things that are said and done by participants in a particular interaction;
2. *Relations*: the relationships between various participants in the interaction (including those who actively participate, those who may be addressed but do not speak, and those who are observing the interaction);
3. *Subject positions*: the roles or positions that people can occupy in a particular interactional setting.

He goes on to discuss ways in which discourse both reflects and influences power relations in communities of practice and societies at large, referring here to the 'power behind discourse'. One of these mechanisms involves restrictions on *access* to particular discourse types. These restrictions are not generally imposed deliberately and directly on particular individuals by more powerful individuals, but are (in effect) built into established systems and conventions that can be very difficult for individuals to challenge. In many professional–client contexts, the person in the professional role is expected to have particular qualifications, credentials or licence to enable him or her to fill the professional role in such encounters. Even when no formal qualifications are required, the fact that people need to be 'apprenticed' into discourses (as we discussed in Chapter 6) means that 'outsiders' with limited experience in the particular features of the discourse in question are unlikely to be able to gain mastery of it.

In looking at the way in which power manifests itself in communication in healthcare settings, we need to keep two further points in mind. The first is that power is not always a negative, oppressive or repressive concept, although it certainly can be in some instances. Naturally, different observers will often disagree in their interpretations of situations where power is a factor, but what is important is to make clear on what basis we are making such interpretations or judgements. The second point is that it is often an oversimplification to talk in terms of 'powerful' and 'powerless' participants in an interaction. Different participants may hold different types of power simultaneously, and the power balance may shift between them over time.

Reflective learning 11.4: Power relations

Consider French and Raven's different 'types' (or bases) of power presented above.

- Which people in your own professional workplace settings exercise the various types of power we list and discuss above?
- Do you think that some individuals exercise more than one type of power simultaneously? How is this exercised and demonstrated?

In Interaction 11.1, it seems clear that Liz (the specialist) is the most 'powerful' person in this interaction. She has *positional* (*legitimate*) power by virtue of her formal designation as a specialist in emergency medicine as well as clinical expertise that her students are (presumably) eager to benefit from. Her power in this interaction can therefore be described as *expert* power as well. Liz's approach to teaching seems engaging and dynamic, and for students who see her as a role model, there may well be a degree of *referent* power as well. This is impossible to determine from the short discourse extract here, but observations of Liz's interactions with students over a longer period of time would help to confirm whether or not this was the case. Finally, to the extent that Liz has the capacity to offer praise and perhaps even positive formal evaluations, there may be an element of *reward* power operating here as well.

In this clinical teaching setting, features of the interaction illustrate Fairclough's notions of 'constraints and controls' on content, relations and subject positioning. From a *content* perspective, we see that Liz selects and sets up the hypothetical scenario (lines 1–2) and then nominates one of the students (May) to respond to it, using questions (lines 2 and 10). It appears that May accepts Liz's moves to 'control' her contributions; as noted above, she does not take offense at the joke that Liz makes at her expense, but laughs and moves quickly to reformulate her response. This could be seen as an acceptance (on the part of May) of Liz's right to control (or guide) the content of her answer given the legitimate and expert power that she holds.

In terms of the *relational* constraints, we see that the 'teacher–student' power relationship between the participants determines what each of the participants is 'allowed' to do and say in this interaction. Once again, we can find evidence in the discourse. As the teacher, Liz (as noted above) controls the topic of the interactions, and also exerts control over turn-taking (allocating turns to a particular speaker). All participants are allowed to ask questions, but Liz asks 'testing' questions to prompt the students (specifically May) to display their knowledge and ways of approaching a situation. When Rob asks a question (line 22), it is to check his own understanding of something that Liz has explained. We would not ordinarily expect either Rob or May in this kind of interaction to ask Liz 'testing' questions (i.e. questions to which they already know the answers).

Finally, power is manifest through the *social positions* or roles that each of the participants adopts. As the most powerful participant, Liz actually 'allocates' a hypothetical role to May at the beginning of the discussion ('OK so you're the resident, May ...', line 1). May is thus playing two roles in this discussion: her 'real' self as a medical student and her 'hypothetical' self as a resident medical officer. Liz adopts the role of the teacher, and in line 18 she also positions herself as someone with experience occupying the specialist-on-call role, advising the students on how to present clinical information.

In the way that Liz guides the students through this hypothetical clinical situation, we can see that she is not only sharing her clinical knowledge, she is also explicitly teaching Rob and May how to manage one of the discourse events that they will face when they become residents. She does this by prompting May (in lines 4–5) to remember that managing this patient's condition is not only about 'doing' (e.g. arranging an MRI scan) but also about 'talking' (contacting the specialist-on-call). Furthermore, she provides advice on *how* to talk to the specialist (lines 17–21). In other words, Liz is providing explicit input in an attempt to help her student to 'access' this type of discourse so that they can, with considerable practice, learn to manage it at an expert level.

11.4   Ethical dilemmas

All human interaction, including the interaction involved in human research, has ethical dimensions. However, 'ethical conduct' is more than simply doing the right thing. It involves acting in the right spirit, out of an abiding respect and concern for one's fellow creatures (National Health and Medical Research Council, Australia 2007).

Healthcare is an area in which ethical dilemmas inevitably arise. Our focus here is not on what does or does not constitute appropriate ethical conduct for healthcare practitioners and personnel, but on the way in which ethical dilemmas are managed interactionally. The word 'dilemma' implies that there is not a single obvious solution on which all parties agree, but that there are different possible positions or courses of action that carry potential ethical consequences. In the area of healthcare practice, it is generally not sufficient to debate and discuss these dilemmas; one is often faced with a situation which requires that a decision be reached as an 'outcome' of this debate and discussion.

11.4.1   Discourse as a focus for discussion

Interaction 11.3

Members of a teaching hospital research ethics committee are reviewing an ethics application for a medical research project, as part of a meeting in which they review the ethical aspects of a number of such projects. The following sequence begins midway through the review, and involves a discussion of the way in which the researchers plan to obtain informed consent from potential participants.

1 Peter:	so how do they get consent from the patients um (.) who asks
2	them?
3 Paul:	the doctor does (.) look on page 6, um, it says [*reading*] 'at the
4	first follow-up appointment the treating doctor will explain the
5	study and obtain consent to use the patient's MRI scans and de-
6	identified clinical details for the purposes of the research'
7 Peter:	so the doctor just gets consent on the spot?
8 Claire:	so it seems yes
9 Peter:	well that's <u>clearly</u> coercive (.) I mean who's going to say no?
10 Jane:	I think they need at least to have a chance to take the
11	information away and read it (.) when <u>I</u> see a doctor there's
12	often so much to process and I can't imagine trying to read this
13	form on the spot and make any kind of informed decision.
14 Paul:	Why not get the research assistant to approach the patients?
15	Take the treating doctor out of the equation altogether?
16 Claire:	I suppose it gives the study some legitimacy if their doctor
17	explains it, perhaps that's what they're thinking (.) but I take
18	your point, the perception of coercion is something that they
19	don't seem to have thought through. So what I suggest we can
20	do is um point this out to the applicants and ask <u>them</u> to
21	suggest ways of minimising the um (.) potential for coercion.
22	We can also put Jane's point to them about um the need to give
23	patients time to read and digest the information rather than
24	springing it on them. Does that sound OK?
25 Others:	[*nods and signals of agreement*]
26 Claire:	OK (.) now with their response when it comes back, is everybody
27	um happy for me to look at it and make a decision, or do we want
28	to discuss it at the next meeting?

Reflective learning 11.5: Power in teams

Look at the committee discussion in Interaction 11.3.

- Who is the leader (chair, in this case) of the committee? How can you tell from the interaction? At what point does it become evident who is chairing the meeting?
- What are the backgrounds of the committee members - are there any clues in the discourse?
- How is power distributed in this interaction, and what evidence for this can you find in the short interaction above?

In this interaction, Peter is a cardiologist, Paul is a clinical psychologist, Claire is a clinical nurse specialist in oncology, and Jane is a community representative on the committee. While you may have been able to identify the community representative from her contribution, the professions of the other participants are not readily evident from the interaction above. The committee represented here (which includes other participants who do not speak at this particular point in the interaction) is another example of a community of practice.

What is interesting is that the members of this committee are *not* making clinical decisions based on their particular specialist knowledge, but are assessing the ethical aspects of a proposed medical research project. In being part of this committee, they are asked to develop a new type of expertise: a familiarity with the 'principles' of ethical research, and an ability to apply a combination of their professional and life experiences to the assessment of research projects that may (at times) fall well outside their specific professional arenas. This challenges traditional power structures and hierarchies (for example between nurses and doctors, or between 'insiders' and 'outsiders' in the healthcare system) and can sometimes result in much flatter power structures. Another way of seeing it is that the holder of 'expert power' shifts between members of the committee as different points are raised throughout the course of the meeting. For example, questions about the potential for a piece of research to produce psychological distress among participants would place the clinical psychologist in the 'expert' role.

Interaction 11.3 also highlights a different sort of leadership style, based strongly on *consensus*. Although Claire is the chair of the committee, this does not become evident until she 'recapitulates' the discussion and proposes a course of action to the other committee members. She then asks the committee if they would like to review the response from the applicants, or whether they are happy to delegate the task of making a decision to the chair.

Reflective learning 11.6: Consensus building

Consider an interaction in which you have been involved where there was a
need to reach a consensus position.

- Was a 'way forward' ultimately decided upon? If not, what do
  you think were the possible reasons for this?
- Did all members of the group appear comfortable with the
  consensus reached? If not, how was this managed by the
  various participants?
- Was there a person who 'led' the discussion (either formally
  designated, or not)? If so, how did he or she approach the role?

11.4.2   Discourse as focus for discussion

Interaction 11.4

Rudi is the Nursing Unit Manager at a small regional hospital. Alison is a general practitioner with a
community practice who also provides medical care for inpatients at the hospital. They are
discussing Mrs Nelson, a 98-year-old woman whose physical condition is very frail, but who has no
cognitive impairment and takes an interest in her own medical condition.

1 Rudi:	Mrs Nelson's son was going to talk to you (.) did he?
2 Alison:	yes, he did (.) he was adamant that I should not tell his mother
3	about the new mass that we found on her CT
4 Rudi:	mm (.) he's been saying the same to us
5 Alison:	I mean I know that there's nothing we can do about it anyway,
6	given her frail condition, but I just feel it's unethical to deceive
7	her
8 Rudi:	mm I know (.) but um (.) just playing devil's advocate for a
9	moment though, perhaps her son feels it'd be unethical to
10	distress //her
11 Alison:	//dist//ress her mm yeah he probably does, and well, he's
12	got a point I have to say (.) I don't think, I mean, we can't lie to her
13	about it, so I suppose it'll come down to how we talk about it
14	with her (.) let me think about it and talk to her son again, and
15	we'll go from there (.) he's a great support to her and I don't
16	want to get him off side
17 Rudi:	Right (.) let me know if I can help or if you'd like me to come
18	along

From Interactions 11.3 and 11.4, we can observe a number of features that characterise the ways that people in healthcare professions – in both formally constituted committees and less formally constituted teams – work through ethical dilemmas. These include:

- posing questions and providing answers aimed at understanding the issue at hand (e.g. the researchers' proposed method of obtaining consent, or the son's position that his elderly mother should not be told about an abnormality on a CT scan);
- expressing personal views on, or reactions to the ethical issues raised, which may be bald and unhedged ('well that's clearly coercive') or expressed in more hedged or tentative terms ('I just feel it's unethical to deceive her');
- presenting the 'other side' of the argument to highlight the dilemma, without expressing overt agreement or disagreement:
  - 'just playing devil's advocate for a moment ...';
  - 'I suppose it gives the study some legitimacy if their doctor explains it, perhaps that's what they're thinking';
- partial solutions or ways forward:
  - 'I think they need to have a chance to take the information away ...';
  - 'Why not get the research assistant to explain the study?';
  - 'So what we can do is ...';
  - 'I suppose it'll come down to how we talk about it ...';
  - 'Let me think about it and talk to her son again and we'll go from there'.

The key points to note for the purposes of our discussion is that dealing with ethical dilemmas is not as simple as each participant 'chipping in' their view and perhaps agreeing or disagreeing with the views of others. While such a format might work in (for instance) a television or radio panel discussion, the institutional context means that a decision or 'way forward' generally needs to emerge from the interaction. At times, individuals may have very strongly held views on particular ethical issues, which will affect the degree to which they can participate in a discussion towards a consensus position. If their view does not ultimately prevail, they may (perhaps appropriately) decide to remove or distance themselves from the process altogether.

Wodak, Kwon and Clarke (2011) identify five discursive strategies that leaders use in the process of building consensus. They characterise these strategies as follows:

1. *Bonding.* This strategy serves to construct a group identity which in turn can motivate the group to reach a consensus position. It is realised linguistically through the use of 'inclusive language', which includes (for instance) greater use

of 'we' and correspondingly less use of 'I'. If you compare Liz (in Interaction 11.1) with Claire (Interaction 11.3) and Alison (Interaction 11.4) in their use of 'we', it becomes evident that 'consensus building' is more salient in some interactions than in others.

2. *Encouraging*. This strategy involves prompting or eliciting the participation of others on the topic under discussion. Linguistically, it is enacted through questions such as 'What do others think?' or 'What do you think, Neil?' or general moves to open up the floor, e.g. 'Can we discuss this now?'

3. *Directing*. This is (in some respects) the opposite of 'encouraging' in that it aims to 'bring the discussion toward closure and resolution by reducing the equivocality of ideas' (Wodak et al. 2011: 605). This can be achieved through direct and overt moves to close down the discussion (e.g. 'We really need to move on, so can you e-mail me any further points, and I'll put together a joint response next week'). It can also be done in a more subtle manner, for instance by summarising the discussion and suggesting a way forward (as Claire does in Interaction 11.3).

4. *Modulating*. This strategy involves adjusting perceptions of urgency and need for decisions/actions so as to achieve optimal outcomes. It aims to convey sufficient urgency to move the interaction forward to a decision (rather than an open-ended discussion), but not stifle deliberation and debate by imposing excessive constraints.

5. *(Re)committing*. This involves moving from a consensus position on an issue to a commitment to action to address it. According to Wodak et al. (2011: 606) it involves 'shifting the frame' to one which involves promises of future action (usually from the chair or leader of the group), or which reminds those present of the group's obligation to act. The 'directing' moves discussed above actually progress seamlessly to statements of commitment (e.g. 'and I'll put together a joint response next week').

Reflective learning 11.7: Ethical dilemmas

Reflect now on your own professional practice:

- What ethical dilemmas do you think are commonly encountered? Do any of the discourse features that we have discussed here (or in earlier chapters) explain how these dilemmas are worked through? Try if you can to note down some examples to illustrate your answer.
- Can you think of an instance in which a consensus position could not be reached by a group that you were a part of? Which (if any) particular discourse strategies employed by the 'chair' or group leader, or by other members, might help to explain why an outcome was not achieved?

11.5   Summary

In this chapter, we have examined some of the ways that contrasting styles of leadership can be enacted from an interactional or discourse perspective. We have also considered ways in which different types of power are manifest through discourse. Finally, we have looked at the process of consensus building that is an important process in many areas of team-based healthcare practice, including the need for teams to grapple with ethical dilemmas that inevitably arise. The following chapter will draw together all of the themes covered in this book, and will shift the focus to the activities, interactions and professional relationships in your own professional life. We will suggest ways of integrating this new learning with your prior knowledge, experience and clinical expertise so that you can apply it effectively in your own professional practice.

12   Ways Forward: Applying Theory to your Practice

Concepts to be introduced, explored and applied

- Making learning relevant
- Exploring communication in your own workplace
- Developing a framework to consolidate learning

Objectives of this chapter
After completing the study of this chapter you will be able to:

- understand the concepts of motivational and practical relevancies;
- make further application of discourse concepts to your own practice experiences;
- develop and apply a total situation focused (TSF) framework to consolidate learning.

12.1   Introduction

In this concluding chapter, we aim to help consolidate your learning and ensure that the discourse concepts we have addressed throughout the book will be relevant to your practice. To achieve this, it is useful to draw on two related concepts: the distinction between what we can call *motivational relevance* and *practical relevance*. These concepts will help you address the key 'so what?' question all practitioners ask: 'so ... I've read through this book, I've grappled with new concepts, I've engaged in reflection activities based on extracts of discourse; but how do they relate to what I do in my daily professional practice?

And if they do relate, does applying them add value to my practice? Are my relationships with the patients I care for, their families and colleagues, enriched; are my practice activities safer, more sensitive and more meaningful?' Asking those questions really depends on the main issue addressed by this book: 'Is this new learning *relevant* to my everyday professional practice?' The questions above are just some of the ones which come to mind. Perhaps you can think of others.

What we want to do in this final chapter is to begin by exploring what we mean by 'relevance' before engaging in another reflection activity. This time, however, you won't be thinking about the questions *we* have posed. We hope you will be posing your own questions as you construct a framework focused on the *total* situation (much as you did in Chapter 1 when we were discussing the concept of total situation focused learning), reinforcing for you the importance/relevance of applying theory to practice. This will help to consolidate not only what you have learned, but also identify what else you want and need to learn, and how you can find ways to address further questions you will surely come up with. No one book can address all the discourse concepts in the world!

12.2   Exploring relevance

In this book, you have worked towards understanding how you can enrich the social and professional practice of healthcare through communicating effectively with others in an environment in which you are intensely engaged. This is no simplistic approach to learning. If it were, it would do a disservice to what you already know from the lived experience of your everyday life: your social and professional/clinical experiences and the relationships that result from them. How you approach, analyse and deal with clinical situations is grounded in your professional knowledge and your experience of similar past situations. You not only engage in professional education and preparation for practice programmes, but you are constantly learning from experiences, building on prior learning and practice situations in your aim to become expert practitioners. As we have tried to emphasise in this book, how you manage your discourse is one such area of practice within your professional field, one in which we all need to develop our discourse to the point where we can become expert discourse practitioners (see Chapter 9). Just as with areas of clinical practice where theory and practice are inextricably and intricately intertwined, so it is the case with making links between theory and method of discourse in the different social situations of practice. These social situations include the myriad healthcare settings and contexts in which health issues arise, and are grappled with, as you seek to find ways of coping with the challenges of healthcare practice. To manage this you are *always* utilising all the tools provided by your understanding of medical science and your own unique professional knowledge base.

What is important, however, is to make the information *motivationally relevant* (see Sarangi and Candlin 2001)in your own engagement with problem solving in specific situations, and in your interactions with other members of the healthcare team (and here we include the patient as a member of the team). In this way, the information that each person has – whether patient or professional carer – is made significant and relevant to others. This involves you recognising the different knowledge bases of your colleagues, and making clear and obvious to them your own disciplinary knowledge base. At the same time, you need to acknowledge the unique knowledge base of patients. It is not just a question of making your professional knowledge motivationally relevant to the situation you are engaged in. That is only a part of the action. It is a matter of making your knowledge motivationally relevant to others in the team, allowing them to make their knowledge motivationally relevant to everyone's situated understanding. Discourse is the route along which we travel to generate and share these understandings. Revisiting Chapter 1 and its discussions and tasks is a good way to return to this, in particular the discussion there of discourse strategies: 'how and what' we say to our interlocutors, and how we interpret and understand what others say to us according to the individual differences of interlocutors in different contexts. The key point here is that the discourse which expresses motivational relevance is socially and culturally determined (see reference to matters of culture in Section 1.2) and is reflected in the local context of the interactions. But to give explanatory value to the text, we need to subject the discourse to analysis. The examples provided in Chapters 1, 2, 3, 6 and 9 show the importance of this analysis. So, we can say that our knowledge of communication and professional relationships is enhanced by an understanding of three key factors. Our central focus is a communication event taking place in a *specific site*. In the context of this book the site is focused on healthcare situations. The three interrelated factors are:

1. our *analysis of discourse*, in particular drawing on aspects of Conversation Analysis, but also the use of metaphor in communication, in constructing coherence in and across conversations;
2. our understanding of *institution(s) and their culture*, specifically here the multidisciplinary nature of healthcare; but we must (i) recognise that culture is not just defined by ethnicity and (ii) recall that institutions are defined both by profession and by bureaucratic institutions, because here the overall institution of healthcare as well as its practices are reflected in the local institution;
3. our awareness of *social theory* incorporating our understanding of how power and ethics impact on particular social situations with their roles and responsibilities, and communities of practice.

These interrelated factors are summarised in Figure 12.1.

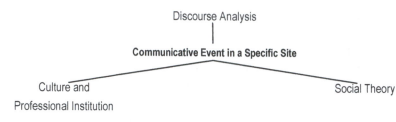

Figure 12.1   The communicative event enhanced by three interrelated factors

12.3   Discourse and social theory

The relevance of discourse to our understanding of the social is highlighted especially in the work of the French sociologist Pierre Bourdieu, specifically in his writings *In other words*: *Essays towards a reflexive sociology* (Bourdieu 1990). Here Bourdieu identifies and defines his three concepts of *habitus*, *field* and *capital*.

Looking first at the construct of 'field', in commenting on Bourdieu, Johnson (1993: 6) suggests that 'field' is 'any social formation ... structured by way of a hierarchically organised series of fields (the economic field, the educational field, the political field, the cultural field etc. ...)'. And here we can add the field of healthcare, which, along with all other fields, has its own conventions concerning its functioning and its relationships of force which are quite independent of those of politics and the economy. What is particularly relevant to us is Johnson's view that '[i]ts structure at any given moment, is determined by the relations between the positions the agents occupy in the field. A field is a dynamic concept in that a change in agents' positions necessarily entails a change in the field's structure' (Johnson 1993: 6).

You have been implicitly drawing on this concept of *field* in your reflective learning activities.

Reflective learning 12.1: Management structures

Consider your own work situation and whether the structure of the organisation is determined by the position held by personalities within the management structure.

- If personalities determine the organisation's structure, how is it reflected in your daily discourse activities with team members and patients? For example, is the managerial approach always 'top down' and autocratic?

(cont.)

Reflective learning 12.1 (cont.)

- How does this structure affect your relations with each other, and how are these relationships illustrated in your discourse? Or is the decision-making, and thus the power, shared amongst all levels of the workforce?

Now look again at Interaction 8.2, between Giovanni and his supervisor.

- What evidence can you discern in the discourse that the decision-making in the management structure is shared? How might the breaking of bad news in this instance compare with how news is delivered in an organisation which takes a top-down approach to management?

Turning now to Bourdieu's second construct, that of *habitus*, Bourdieu offers the following definition:

> The source of historical action, that of the artist, the scientist, or the member of government just as much as that of the worker or that of the petty civil servant, is not an active subject confronting society as if that society were an object constituted externally. The source resides neither in consciousness nor in things but in the relationship between two stages of the social, that is between the history objectified in things, in the form of the institutions, and history incarnated in bodies, in that form of enduring dispositions which I call habitus (Bourdieu 1990: 190).

In their commentaries on the work of Bourdieu, Taylor (1993) and Johnson (1993) emphasise how habitus influences all aspects of our communication with others when they write:

> a system of durable transposable dispositions ... A bodily disposition is a habitus when it encodes a certain cultural understanding. The habitus in this sense ... always has an expressive dimension. It gives expression to certain meanings that things and people have for us, and it is precisely by giving such expressions that these meanings exist for us ... (Taylor 1993: 58).

> [T]he habitus is sometimes described as 'the feel for the game', a 'practical sense' ... that inclines agents to act and react in specific situations in a manner that is not always calculated and that is not simply a question of conscious obedience to rules. Rather, it is a set of dispositions that generates practices and perceptions. The habitus is the result of a long process

of inculcation, beginning in early childhood, which becomes a 'second sense' or a second nature. According to Bourdieu's definition, the dispositions represented by the habitus are 'durable' in that they last through an agent's lifetime. They are 'transposable' in that they may generate practices in multiple and diverse fields of activity, and they are 'structured structures', in that they inevitably incorporate the objective social conditions of their inculcation (Johnson 1993: 5).

Bourdieu's writings and these commentaries encourage us to see our professional selves as inhabiting a physical and psychological body that is steeped in a history developed over many years. Not only is our professional knowledge acquired over time, but also our values, beliefs and behaviours – cultural understandings – are progressively developed; this knowledge and cultural understanding influence and impact on the presentation of our professional selves. We think, act, speak like a doctor, nurse, physiotherapist, social worker, etc. because we *are* a doctor, nurse, physiotherapist, social worker, etc. We are what we are and are seen and considered by others for what we are. We have certain expectations of ourselves because of our *habitus*, just as others have expectations of our behaviours. We talk and behave, and others expect us to talk and behave, as health professionals because we *are* health professionals. In Bourdieu's words, we are in a dialectic relationship with an objective event – our surroundings, our professional world. He extends his analysis by arguing that each person brings to the event what he terms *capital*, not in any Marxist sense, but as capital (we might even say *resources*) which is in non-material form – cultural, symbolic and social. Such capital, Bourdieu believes, is seen always as a means of exerting power. (Here you might wish to reflect on the discussion in Chapter 11 where we presented the work of French and Raven and their discussion of the notion of types of power.) As Bourdieu writes:

> These fundamental social powers are, according to my empirical investigations, firstly *economic* capital, in its various kinds; secondly *cultural* capital or better, *informational* capital, again in its various kinds; and thirdly two forms of capital which are strongly correlated, *social* capital, which consists of resources based on connections and group membership and *symbolic* capital, which is the form different types of capital take once they are perceived and recognised as legitimate (Bourdieu, cited in Calhoun 1993: 70).

Within any healthcare situation, you are first and foremost concerned with *informational (cultural) capital*, since competent professional practice demands a sound knowledge base not usually available to patients; but secondly, and equally, you are engaged with *social capital*, where healthcare professionals exercise authority over patients, perhaps excluding them from discussions of their condition. You might consider that *symbolic capital*, represented by the artefacts of your professional practice (e.g., tools for assessing health needs, equipment for administering therapies), is also a factor which indicates differences not only between professional and patient, but between professional groups. These forms of capital then represent differences which are at once a source of separation (of patient from healthcare professional, and health professional from health professional), but also a means of unity when each form of capital is used cooperatively to achieve a common purpose – the delivery of healthcare. As such, you could see healthcare practitioners and patients as a group within the bureaucratic institution, and then expect to see instances of alignment and affiliation as agents (i.e. carers and patients) display in their discourse their affiliations and different alignments (see particularly the discourse processes in turn-taking, topic exchange, coherence, facework, for example in Chapters 2, 3, 4 and 10).

The question now arises of how you adapt your discourse to the different healthcare contexts and specialty areas. How does your *habitus* affect your behaviours? How might your discourse change according to the professional roles you undertake within that specialty area? If you are undertaking a patient-education role, is your discourse qualitatively different from when you are engaged in research activity, or within a case conference with colleagues? It is worth spending some time reflecting on these questions, because how you respond to these questions is fundamental to the way you interact with others and how you engage in professional practice activities.

Reflective learning 12.2: Discourse and organisational structures

In your professional practice, consider your relationships with colleagues from other healthcare disciplines.

- What differences can you identify according to the person/s you are relating to (colleague or patient) and their individual differences? (Here you might wish to refer to Chapter 1 and the World of Communication model.) What considerations do you make to ensure that your professional and discourse goals are achieved?
- Reflect on your practice and identify some of the roles you adopt in your workplace. How do they differ according to the clinical situation and the specialty area of practice?
  - What discourse demands do the different roles make on your interactions?
  - Within those roles, reflect on your discourse. How does it change according to the role you are engaged in?

12.4   Developing frameworks

One of the main objectives of this chapter (indeed we could say the *main* objective) is to ensure that your learning is *motivationally relevant*. One way of ensuring that is to construct a *framework* within which you can reflect on and place your learning from your studies in this book. Such a framework helps you to make relevant your own learning and at the same time helps you to reveal those areas and those themes where you want/need to learn more.

In Chapter 1 we posed questions which formed the basis of all your reflective learning activities; now we will extend and adapt them in light of what you have learned so far through the readings and reflection activities.

The questions we asked were:

- What do I know about: (a) the professional issues presented in clinical situations and (b) the communication issues that might arise in different contexts?
- From my own accumulated life/professional experiences and body of knowledge, what do I already know about the work, lives and health situations of the colleagues and patients involved in specific clinical scenarios?
- What do I need to know about this particular healthcare situation so that outcomes are achieved?
- How will I determine the appropriate discourse strategies so that the communication issues I have identified are relevant to my own workplace? How in fact can my discourse be integrated with my clinical knowledge to achieve desired outcomes?

It is these questions that will help guide your reflections as you determine what you have learned and understood from your readings, and how you ensure your knowledge is relevant to your practice. Frameworks are an effective and useful visual way of sorting out and organising your thoughts about what you have learned. For example, as you have worked through the book, you will have thought not only about what you have read, but, in your reflections, thoughts might have come to you that are tangential to the main theme. You may have been led to read other papers, you may have been reminded of experiences that on the surface are not directly related to your reflections, but nevertheless have informed your practice as questions in your mind have been 'triggered' which your natural curiosity wished to explore further so that your learning and your clinical practice is enhanced. It is these processes that a framework can help visualise.

Here we offer our thoughts on developing a framework which considers the total situation: the social, emotional, physical and pathophysiological as it is reflected in the discourses of care. Such an approach can both make your learning motivationally relevant and consolidate it, if you draw from your clinical practice a specific experience and allow your accumulated knowledge – old and knew – to extend your learning so that ideas are generated which will change practice. As we have seen in this book, these may be discourse practices used in the clinical setting, thus integrating the two areas of healthcare practice and discourse practice. As an example, we might take the health situation of a man with a neurological condition to construct our framework. We will consider the total situation in our development of a framework related to such a patient and in our response to his condition we will keep in mind:

- *our knowledge* (what we already know about the person: the disease pathology, the effects of the diagnosis: physically, emotionally, socio-economically, spiritually on the person, significant others, professional health carers and the institution; our *previous experiences* of the patient, professional health carers and significant others, and available resources;
- our *identified goals* (short, medium, long term);
- what we *need to know* (e.g. about the patient, the disease and its trajectory, the contribution of other healthcare team members);
- *the resources* available to us, human and material, that will inform our knowledge base and constrain or promote our professional actions.

Our aim is to develop a total situation focused framework (TSF framework). We will take as our focus a patient, Mr Smith. As you reflect on his situation you will be drawing on previous knowledge accumulated from everyday life and clinical experiences. You will also be drawing upon your theoretical knowledge obtained from professional education studies as well as your current learning experience presented in this book and related readings. What you will be engaged in is a process of integration of past and present learning experiences so that they can be applied to a clinical situation resulting in a TSF framework of care for a specific person with specific needs and in a specific situation. This will enhance your knowledge base and, importantly, inform your practice.

Reflective learning activity 12.3: The focal situation

Mr Smith is 56 years old and has been admitted for respite care because his wife has been admitted to hospital for major surgery. Their 18-year-old son is in his first year of a bachelor degree course and is unable to undertake the complex care necessary to meet the needs of his father who has secondary progressive multiple sclerosis.

(cont.)

Reflective learning activity 12.3 (cont.)

Using your prior and new knowledge you could develop a *framework* which will:

- allow you to explore and identify
  - what you know of Mr Smith's total health situation,
  - what you need to know to identify his needs,
  - what actions you will need to take to gain more knowledge,
  - what discourse concepts are triggered in your mind,
  - where you will go to find more information;
- trigger other thoughts in your mind which are not identified here and which will need to address to enlarge your knowledge in your quest for expertise so that you can provide expert individualised appropriate and sensitive care.

12.4.1 An example of a TSF framework

You may use the example shown in Figure 12.2 to construct your own TSF framework and/ or apply it to other clinical situations.

Note: this is *our* version of such a framework. The items and words which we have identified are just examples for you to add to and subtract from as appropriate for you. Indeed you are encouraged to make your own links according to your learning needs in specific situations, and to 'fit' the way *your* mind works and the development of *your* thought processes. Each word in this framework may trigger other thoughts which you may wish to explore, and of course these triggers may trigger others – the process might seem endless.

12.5   Summary

Now that you have completed this final reflective learning activity, we hope that you will want and be able to approach other situations which you encounter, both in clinical practice and in everyday life, seen through a new lens. Of course, you will not need to apply all that you have learned from your studies and reflections in this book in relation to *all* situations. You will almost certainly encounter situations which have not of necessity been addressed in this book, but importantly you will have developed key skills, which will help you explore unknown areas and engage in novel experiences.

What you will have done in having integrated knowledge acquired from prior and new learning experiences with your everyday life and professional practice experiences is to develop a new gestalt. The final framework is one where you

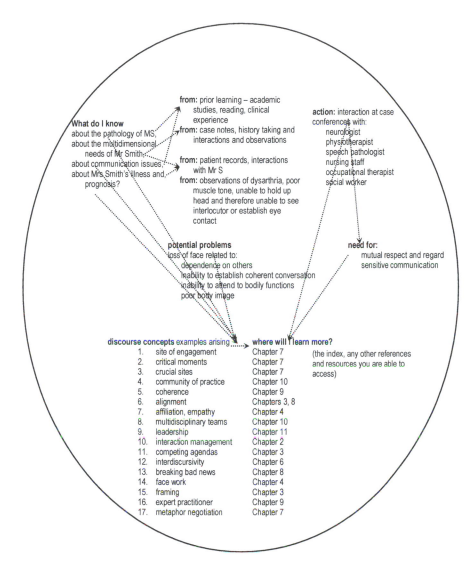

from: prior learning – academic studies, reading, clinical experience
from: case notes, history taking and interactions and observations

What do I know about the pathology of MS, about the multidimensional needs of Mr Smith, about communication issues, about Mrs Smith's illness and prognosis?

from: patient records, interactions with Mr S
from: observations of dysarthria, poor muscle tone, unable to hold up head and therefore unable to see interlocutor or establish eye contact

action: interaction at case conferences with:
   neurologist
   physiotherapist
   speech pathologist
   nursing staff
   occupational therapist
   social worker

potential problems
   loss of face related to:
   dependence on others
   inability to establish coherent conversation
   inability to attend to bodily functions
   poor body image

need for:
   mutual respect and regard
   sensitive communication

discourse concepts examples arising   **where will I learn more?**

1.	site of engagement	Chapter 7
2.	critical moments	Chapter 7
3.	crucial sites	Chapter 7
4.	community of practice	Chapter 10
5.	coherence	Chapter 9
6.	alignment	Chapters 3, 8
7.	affiliation, empathy	Chapter 4
8.	multidisciplinary teams	Chapter 10
9.	leadership	Chapter 11
10.	interaction management	Chapter 2
11.	competing agendas	Chapter 3
12.	interdiscursivity	Chapter 6
13.	breaking bad news	Chapter 8
14.	face work	Chapter 4
15.	framing	Chapter 3
16.	expert practitioner	Chapter 9
17.	metaphor negotiation	Chapter 7

(the index, any other references and resources you are able to access)

Figure 12.2   An example of a TSF framework

have applied your new learning to a clinical situation and by so doing you have revised, established, and gained new theoretical learning. New knowledge and new areas of expertise will contribute to your analysis and understanding of the relationships which occur in the professional workplace. In doing so, you can knowingly make use of your resources of communication strategies to enhance your practice. In this way, you display that you are not solely a member of your own particular clinical profession, but you have also become a health discourse practitioner.

References

Antaki, C. (2011). *Applied conversation analysis: Intervention and change in institutional talk*. Basingstoke: Palgrave Macmillan.

Archer, J. and Coyne, S.M. (2005). An integrated review of indirect, relational, and social aggression. *Personality and Social Psychology Review* 9: 212-30.

Baron-Cohen, S. (2003). *The essential difference: The truth about the male and female brain*. New York: Basic Books.

Barton, E. (2007). Institutional and professional orders of ethics in the discourse practices of research recruitment in oncology. In R. Iedema (ed.), *The discourse of hospital communication: Tracing complexities in contemporary health care organizations*. Basingstoke: Palgrave Macmillan.

Bateson, G. (1955). A theory of play and fantasy. *Psychiatric Research Reports* 2: 39-51

Benner, P. (1984). *From novice to expert: Excellence and power in clinical nursing practice*. Menlo Park: Addison-Wesley Publishing Company.

Bennis, W. (1999). Five competencies of new leaders. *Executive Excellence* 16(7): 4-5.

Bhatia, V.K. (2010). Interdiscursivity in professional communication. *Discourse and Communication* 4(1): 32-50.

Bilbow, G. (1997). Cross-cultural impression management in the multicultural workplace: The special case of Hong Kong. *Journal of Pragmatics* 28(4): 461-87.

Bordage, G. (1994). Elaborated knowledge: A key to successful diagnostic thinking. *Academic Medicine* 69(11): 883-85.

Bourdieu, P. (1990). *In other words: Essays towards a reflexive sociology*, trans. M. Adamson. Cambridge: Polity Press.

Brown, P., and Levinson, S.C. (1987). *Politeness: Some universals in language usage*. Cambridge: Cambridge University Press.

Burke, K. (1945). *A grammar of motives*. New York: Prentice Hall.

Calhoun, C. (1993). Habitus, field and capital: The question of historic specificity. In C. Calhoun, E. LiPuma and M. Postone (eds.), *Bourdieu: Critical perspectives*. Cambridge: Polity Press: 61-88.

Cameron, L. (2010). What is metaphor and why does it matter? In L. Cameron and R. Maslen, *Metaphor analysis: Research practice in applied linguistics, social sciences and the humanities*. London and Oakville: Equinox.

Candlin, C.N. (1997). General editor's introduction. In B.-L. Gunnarsson, P. Linell and B. Nordberg (eds.), *The construction of professional discourse*. London: Longman: viii-xiv.

Candlin C.N. (2010). Engendering trust in healthcare interactions. 2010 Ilana Ruschin Oration, University of Melbourne.

Candlin, C.N. and Crichton J. (2013). *Discourses of trust*. Basingstoke: Palgrave.

Candlin, C.N. and Maley, Y. (1997). Intertextuality and interdiscursivity in the discourse of alternative dispute resolution. In B.-L. Gunnarsson, P. Linell and B. Nordberg (eds.), *The construction of professional discourse*. London: Longman: 201-22.

Candlin, S. (1992). Communication for nurses: Implications for nurse education. *Nurse Education Today* 12: 445-51.

Candlin, S. (1997a). *Towards excellence in nursing: An analysis of the discourse of nurses and patients in the context of health assessments*. Unpublished PhD thesis, University of Lancaster.

Candlin, S. (1997b). Primary health care: Directions for nursing practice and teaching. *Asian Journal of Nursing Studies* 3(1): 15-22.

Candlin, S. (2002). Taking risks: An indicator of nursing expertise? *Research on Language and Social Interaction* 35(2): 173-93.

Candlin, S. (2008). *Therapeutic communication: A lifespan approach*. Sydney: Pearson.

Candlin, S. and Candlin, C. (2007), Nursing through time and space: Some challenges to the construct of the community of practice. In R. Iedema (ed.), *The discourse of hospital communication: Tracing complexities in contemporary health care organizations*. Basingstoke, Hampshire: Palgrave Macmillan: 244-67.

Castells, M. (1990). *The rise of the network society. The information age: economy, society and culture*, Vol. 1, Oxford: Blackwell.

Chafe, W. (1992). The flow of ideas in a sample of written language. In W.C. Mann and S.A. Thompson (eds.), *Discourse description: Diverse linguistic analysis of a fund-raising text*. Amsterdam and Philadelphia: John Benjamins Publishing Company: 267-94.

Coupland, J. (ed.) (2000). *Small talk*. Harlow: Longman.

Coupland, N. and Jaworski, A. (1997). Relevance, accommodation and conversation: Modeling the social dimension of communication. *Multilingua* 16(2-3): 233-58.

Crawford, P. and Brown, B. (2011). Fast healthcare: Brief communication, traps and opportunities. *Patient Education and Counselling* 82: 3-10.

Davis, M. (1994). *Empathy: A social psychological approach*. Madison: Brown and Benchmark.

Drew, P. and Heritage, J. (1992). Analyzing talk at work: an introduction. In P. Drew and J. Heritage (eds.), *Talk at work: Interaction in institutional settings*. Cambridge: Cambridge University Press: 3-65.

Dreyfus, S.E. (1982). Formal models vs. human situational understanding: Inherent limitations on the modelling of business expertise. *Office: Technology and People* 1: 135-55.

Dreyfus, S.E. and Dreyfus, H.L. (1980). A five-stage model of mental activities involved in directed skill acquisitions. Unpublished report supported by the Air Force Office of Scientific Research (AFSC), USAF (Contract F49620-79-C-0063), University of California at Berkley. In P. Benner (1984), *From novice to expert: Excellence and power in clinical nursing practice*. Menlo Park: Addison-Wesley Publishing Company: 13-14.

Dunleavy, K.N., Chory, R.M. and Goodboy, A.K. (2010). Responses to deception in the workplace: Perceptions of credibility, power, and trustworthiness. *Communication Studies* 61(2): 239-55.

Eckert, P. and McConnell-Ginet, S. (1992). Think practically and look locally: Language and gender as community-based practice. *Annual Review of Anthropology* 21: 461-90.

Fairclough, N. (1989). *Language and power*. London: Longman.

Fairclough, N.L. (1992). *Discourse and social change*. Cambridge: Polity Press.

Fairclough, N. (1995). *Critical discourse analysis: The critical study of language*. London: Longman.

Faulkner, A. (1992). *Effective interaction with patients*. Edinburgh: Churchill Livingstone.

French, J., and Raven, B.H. (1959). The bases of social power. In D. Cartwright (ed.), *Studies in social power*. Ann Arbor, MI: Institute for Social Research: 150-67.

Garfinkel, H. (1967). *Studies in ethnomethodology*. Englewood Cliffs, NJ: Prentice Hall.

Glaser, B. and Strauss, A. (1965). *Awareness of dying*. Chicago: Aldine Publishers.

Goffman, E. (1959). *The presentation of self in everyday life*. Garden City, NY: Doubleday.

Goffman, E. (1974). *Frame analysis: An essay on the organization of experience*. Oxford: Blackwell.

Goffman, E. (1981). *Forms of talk*. Philadelphia: University of Pennsylvania Press.

Gumperz, J.J. (1982). *Language and social identity*. New York: Cambridge University Press.

Gumperz, J.J. (1992). Contextualization and understanding. In A. Duranti and C. Goodwin (eds.), *Rethinking context: Language as an interactive phenomenon*. Cambridge: Cambridge University Press: 229-52.

Hak, T. (1999). 'Text' and 'Con-text': Talk bias in studies of health care work. In S. Sarangi and C. Roberts (eds.), *Talk, work, and institutional order: Discourse in medical, mediation and management settings*. Berlin: Mouton de Gruyter: 427-52.

Halpern, J. (1996). Empathy: Using resonance emotions in the service of curiosity. In H.M. Spiro, E. Peschel, M.G. Curnen and D. St. James (eds.),

Empathy and the practice of medicine: Beyond pills and the scalpel. New Haven: Yale University Press: 160-73.

Holmes, J., Schnurr, A., Chan, A. and Chiles, T. (2003). The discourse of nursing leadership. *Te Reo* 46: 31-46.

Hunt, M. (1991). Being friendly and informal: Reflected in nurses', terminally ill patients' and their relatives' conversations at home. *Journal of Advanced Nursing* 16(8): 929-38.

Hutchby, I. (2007). *The discourse of child counselling.* Amsterdam: John Benjamins.

Hutchby, I. and Wooffitt, R. (1998). *Conversation analysis.* Cambridge: Polity Press.

Iedema, R. (ed.) (2007). *The discourse of hospital communication: Tracing complexities in contemporary health care organizations.* Basingstoke: Palgrave Macmillan.

Iedema, R. and Scheeres, H. (2003). From doing work to talking work: Renegotiating knowing, doing and identity. *Applied Linguistics* 24(3): 316-37.

Jefferson, G. (1972). Side sequences. In D. Sudnow (ed), *Studies in social interaction.* New York: Free Press.

Johnson, R. (ed.) (1993). *The field of cultural production.* Cambridge: Polity Press.

Jones, R. (1996). *Responses to AIDS awareness discourse: A cross-cultural frame analysis.* Research Monograph 10. Hong Kong: City University of Hong Kong.

Kendon, A. (1992). *Conducting interaction: Patterns of focused encounters.* Cambridge: Cambridge University Press.

Kerosuo, H. (2007). Renegotiating disjunctions in interorganizationaly provided care. In R. Iedema (ed.), *The discourse of hospital communication: Tracing complexities in contemporary health care organizations.* Basingstoke: Palgrave Macmillan: 138-60.

Kitzinger, C. (2011). Working with childbirth helplines: The contributions and limitation of Conversational Analysis. In C. Antaki (ed.), *Applied Conversational Analysis: Intervention and change in institutional talk.* Basingstoke: Palgrave Macmillan.

Lakoff, R. (1973). The logic of politeness, or minding your P's and Q's. In C. Corum, T.C. Smith-Stark and A. Weiser (eds.), *Papers from the Ninth Regional Meeting of the Chicago Linguistics Society.* Chicago: Chicago Linguistics Society: 292-305.

Lakoff, R. (1975). *Language and woman's place.* New York: Harper and Row.

Lave, J. and Wenger, E. (1991). *Situated learning: Legitimate peripheral participation.* Cambridge: Cambridge University Press.

Lawler, J. (1991). *Behind the screens.* Melbourne: Churchill Livingstone.

Leaper, C. and Robnett, R.D. (2011). Women are more likely than men to use tentative language, aren't they? A meta-analysis testing for gender differences and moderators. *Psychology of Women Quarterly* 35(1): 129-42.

Levinson, S. (1983). *Pragmatics*. Cambridge: Cambridge University Press.

Levinson, S.C. (1988). Putting linguistics on a proper footing: Explorations in Goffman's participation framework. In P. Drew, and A. Wootton (eds.), *Goffman: Exploring the interaction order*. Oxford: Polity Press: 161-227.

Linell, P. (1998). Discourse across boundaries: On recontextualizations and the blending of voices in professional discourse. *Text* 18(2): 143-57.

Lipovsky, C. (2006). Candidates' negotiation of their expertise in job interviews. *Journal of Pragmatics* 38(8): 1147-74.

Luk, J. (2010). Talking to score: Impression management in L2 oral assessment and the co-construction of a test discourse genre. *Language Assessment Quarterly* 7(1): 25-53.

Lum, M. and Fitzgerald, A. (2007). Dialogues for negotiating priorities in unplanned emergency surgical queues. In R. Iedema (ed.), *The discourse of hospital communication: Tracing complexities in contemporary health care organizations*. Basingstoke: Palgrave Macmillan: 90-108.

Lutfey, K. and Maynard, D.W. (1998). Bad news in oncology: How physician and patient talk about death and dying without using those words. *Social Psychology Quarterly* 61(4): 321-41.

MacDonald, M.L. (1978). Measuring assertion: A model and method. *Behaviour Therapy* 9: 889-99.

Maguire S., Phillips N. and Hardy C. (2001). When 'silence = death', keep talking: Trust, control and the discursive construction of identity in the Canadian HIV/AIDS Treatment Domain. *Organisation Studies* 22 (2): 285-310.

Markee, N. (2000). *Conversation analysis*. Mahwah, NJ: Lawrence Erlbaum Associates.

Maynard, D.W. (1989). Perspective display sequences in conversation. *Western Journal of Speech Communication* 53: 91-113.

Maynard, D.W. (1992). On clinicians coimplicating recipients' perspective in the delivery of diagnostic news. In P. Drew and J. Heritage (eds.), *Talk at work: Interaction in institutional settings*. Cambridge: Cambridge University Press: 331-58.

Maynard, D.W. (1996). On 'realization' in everyday life: The forecasting of bad news as a social relation. *American Sociological Review* 61: 109-31.

Maynard, D. (1997). The news delivery sequence: bad news and good news in conversational interaction. *Research on Language and Social Interaction* 30(2): 93-130.

Maynard, D. (1998). Praising versus blaming the messenger: Moral issues in deliveries of good news and bad news. *Research on Language and Social Interaction* 1(3-4): 359-95.

National Health and Medical Research Council Australia (2007). *National Statement on Ethical Conduct in Human Research*. Canberra: Australian Government.

O'Grady C (2011a). *The nature of expert communication as required for the General Practice of medicine: A discourse analytical study*. Unpublished PhD thesis, Macquarie University.

O'Grady, C. (2011b). Teaching the communication of empathy in patient-centred medicine. In B. Hoekje and S. Tipton (eds.), *English language and the medical profession: Instructing and assessing the communication skills of international physicians*. Bingley: Emerald Press.

O'Grady, C. and Candlin, C.N. (2013). Engendering trust in a multiparty consultation involving an adolescent patient. In C.N. Candlin and J. Crichton (eds.), *Discourses of trust*. Basingstoke: Palgrave: 57-76.

Pincock, S. (2004). Poor communication lies at the heart of NHS complaints. *British Medical Journal* 328(7430): 10.

Poggi, I. (2005). The goals of persuasion. *Pragmatics and Cognition* 13(2): 297-336.

Pounds, B. (2011). Empathy as 'appraisal': A new language-based approach to the exploration of clinical empathy. *Journal of Applied Linguistics and Professional Practice* 7(2): 145-68.

Ribeiro, B.T. (1996). Conflict talk in psychiatric discharge interview: Struggling between personal and official footings. In C.R. Caldas-Coulthard and M. Coulthard (eds.), *Texts and practices: Readings in critical discourse analysis*. London and New York: Routledge: 179-93.

Roger, P. and Code. C. (2011). Lost in translation: Issues of content validity in interpreter mediated aphasia assessments. *International Journal of Speech-Langauge Pathology* 13(1): 61-73.

Roger, P. and Code, C. (forthcoming). Diverging professional orientations to content and form in interpreter-mediated aphasia assessments. In S. Sarangi (ed.), *Interpreter mediated healthcare consultations*. Sheffield: Equinox.

Ruusuvuori, J. (2005). Comparing homeopathic and general practice consultations: The case of problem presentation. *Communication and Medicine* 2(2): 123-35.

Sacks, H. (1992). *Lectures on conversation*, Vol. 2. Oxford: Blackwell.

Sacks, M., Schegloff, E. and Jefferson, G. (1974). A simplest systematics for the organization of turn taking in conversation. *Language* 50(4): 696-735.

Sarangi, S.K. (1990). *The dynamics of institutional discourse: An intercultural perspective*. Unpublished doctoral thesis, Lancaster University.

Sarangi, S. and Candlin, C.N. (2001). 'Motivational relevancies': Some methodological reflections on social theoretical and sociolinguistic practice. In N. Coupland, S. Sarangi and C.N. Candlin (eds.), *Sociolinguistics and Social Theory*. Harlow: Pearson Education: 350-85.

Sarangi, S. and Roberts, C. (1999). *Talk, work, and institutional order: Discourse in medical, mediation and management settings*. Berlin: Mouton de Gruyter.

Schegloff, E.A. (1972). Notes on conversational practice: Formulating place. In D. Sudnow (ed.) *Studies in social interaction*. New York: The Free Press: 75-119.

Schegloff, E.A (2007). *Sequence organization in interaction: A primer in conversation analysis*. Cambridge: Cambridge University Press.

Schegloff, E.A. and Sacks, H. (1973). Opening up closings. *Semiotica* 8(4): 289-327.

Scheuer, J. (2001). Recontextualization and communicative styles in job interviews. *Discourse Studies* 3(2): 223-48.

Schön, D. (1983). *The reflective practitioner: How professionals think in action*. London: Temple Smith.

Scollon, R. (1998). *Mediated discourse as social interaction: The study of news discourse*. London: Longman.

Scollon, R. (2001). Action and text: Towards an integrated understanding of the place of text in social (inter)action, mediated discourse analysis and the problem of social action. In R. Wodak and M. Meyer (eds.), *Methods of critical discourse analysis*. London: Sage Publications: 139-83.

Sutcliffe, K.M., Lewton, E. and Rosenthal, M.M (2004). Communication failures: An insidious contributor to medical mishaps. *Academic Medicine* 79(2): 186-94.

Talmy, S. (2011). The interview as a collaborative achievement: Interaction, identity, and ideology in a speech event. *Applied Linguistics* 32(1): 25-42.

Tannen, D. (1984). *Coherence in spoken and written discourse*, Vol. 12. Norwood, NJ: Ablex Publishing Corp.

Tannen, D. (1989). *Talking voices: Repetition, dialogue, and imagery in conversational discourse*. Cambridge: Cambridge University Press.

Tannen, D. (1993). What's in a frame? Surface evidence for underlying expectations. In D. Tannen (ed.), *Framing in discourse*. New York: Oxford University Press: 14-56.

Tannen, D. and Wallat, C. (1993). Interactive frames and knowledge schemas in interaction: Examples from a medical examination/interview. In D. Tannen (ed.), *Framing in discourse*. New York: Oxford University Press: 57-76.

Taylor, C. (1993). To follow a rule. In C. Calhoun, E. Li Puma and M. Postone (eds.), *Bourdieu: Critical perspectives*. Cambridge: Polity Press: 45-60.

Thompson, J.B. (1990). *Ideology and modern culture*. Cambridge: Polity Press.

Wadensjö, C. (1998). *Interpreting as interaction*. London: Longman.

Weick, K. and Sutcliffe, K.M. (2001). *Managing the unexpected: Assuring high performance in the age of complexity*. San Fancisco: Jossey-Bass.

Wenger, E. (1998). *Communities of practice: Learning, meaning and identity*. Cambridge: Cambridge University Press.

Wenger, E. (2006). *Communities of practice: A brief introduction.* Retrieved 1 February 2012 from www.ewenger.com/theory.

Wilson, K. and Gallois, C. (1993). *Assertion and its social context.* Oxford: Pergamon Press.

Wittgenstein, L. (1958), *Philosophical investigations*, 2nd edn. Oxford: Blackwell Publishers.

Wodak, R., Kwon, W., and Clarke, I. (2011). Getting people on board: Discursive leadership for consensus building in team meetings. *Discourse and Society* 22(5): 592-644.

Zaleznik, A. (1992). Managers and leaders: Are they different? *Harvard Business Review*, March–April: 126-35.

Index of Authors

Index of Subjects

Lightning Source UK Ltd.
Milton Keynes UK
UKOW07f0825110515

251258UK00001B/3/P